Visual Perception Problems in Children with AD/HD, Autism, and Other Learning Disabilities

also by Lisa A. Kurtz

How to Help a Clumsy Child
Strategies for Young Children with Developmental Motor Concerns
ISBN 1 84310 754 6

of related interest

Seeing Through New Eyes
Changing the Lives of Children with Autism, Asperger Syndrome
and other Developmental Disabilities Through Vision Therapy
Melvin Kaplan
Foreword by Stephen M. Edelson
ISBN 1 84310 800 3

Understanding Sensory Dysfunction
Learning, Development and Sensory Dysfunction in Autism
Spectrum Disorders, ADHD, Learning Disabilities and Bipolar Disorder
Polly Godwin Emmons and Liz McKendry Anderson
ISBN 1 84310 806 2

Sensory Perceptual Issues in Autism and Asperger Syndrome
Different Sensory Experiences – Different Perceptual Worlds
Olga Bogdashina
Forewords by Wendy Lawson and Theo Peeters
ISBN 1 84310 166 1

Sensory Smarts
A Book for Kids with ADHD or Autism Spectrum Disorders
Struggling with Sensory Integration Problems
Kathleen A. Chara and Paul J. Chara, Jr. with Christian P. Chara
Illustrated by J.M. Berns
ISBN 1 84310 783 X

Visual Perception Problems in Children with AD/HD, Autism, and Other Learning Disabilities

A Guide for Parents and Professionals

Lisa A. Kurtz

Jessica Kingsley Publishers
London and Philadelphia

OPTO

ↄ 14845477

First published in 2006
by Jessica Kingsley Publishers
116 Pentonville Road
London N1 9JB, UK
and
400 Market Street, Suite 400
Philadelphia, PA 19106, USA

www.jkp.com

Library of Congress Cataloging in Publication Data
Kurtz, Lisa A.
    Visual perception problems in children with AD/HD, autism and other learning disabilities : a guide for parents and professionals / Lisa A. Kurtz.-- 1st American pbk. ed.
        p. cm.
    Includes bibliographical references and index.
    ISBN-13: 978-1-84310-826-9 (pbk.)
    ISBN-10: 1-84310-826-7 (pbk.)
    1. Attention-deficit hyperactivity disorder. 2. Autism. 3. Autism in children. I. Title.
    RJ506.H9K87 2006
    616.85'89--dc22

                                            2005037054

British Library Cataloguing in Publication Data
A CIP catalogue record for this book is available from the British Library

ISBN-13: 978 1 84310 826 9
ISBN-10: 1 84310 826 7

Printed and bound in Great Britain by
Athenaeum Press, Gateshead, Tyne and Wear

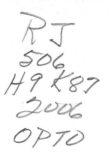
This book is dedicated to the community of learners at Jameson School in Old Orchard Beach, Maine. The energy and enthusiasm of students, staff, and parents are an inspiration! As we continue to work and learn together, may we all come to see more clearly how to promote the best possible outcomes in our special students!

CONTENTS

Introduction   **11**
Importance of vision to learning and development
and the purpose of the book   11

1. **Anatomy and Structure of the Visual System**   **15**
   The eye and extraocular muscles   15
   The optic pathways   18

2. **The Early Development of Visual Skills**   **21**
   Visual skills in the first year of life   21
   Toddlers and preschoolers   23

3. **Do You See What I See? Problems with Visual Skills**   **25**
   Structural vision problems   25
   Functional vision impairments   28
   Visual perception problems   33

4. **Finding Professional Help for Problems with Vision**   **37**
   Warning signs of functional vision and perceptual disorders   38
   Selecting a vision specialist   40
   Assessment of cognitive visual perceptual disorders   48

5. **Activities for Improving Visual Skills**   **61**
   Activities to improve functional vision   62
   Activities to improve visual perception   70

6. **Helping Children to Compensate for Problems with Vision**   **75**
   Strategies for maintaining visual hygiene   75
   Possible compensatory strategies for vision difficulties   76

7.   **Resources**   **79**
Recommended reading   79
Helpful agencies, organizations, and websites   81
Publishers of tests for visual perception   85
Suppliers of therapy and educational materials   86

APPENDIX: EQUIPMENT FABRICATION   89
Balance board   89
One-legged balance stool   90
Finger chart   92

GLOSSARY   95

INDEX   105

List of figures and tables

Figures

1.1	Structure of the eye	16
1.2	Process of accommodation	18
1.3	Visual pathways	19
3.1	Refractive errors	29
3.2	The eye muscles	31
5.1	Clothes hanger paddle	65
5.2	Bottle scoop	65
5.3	Stick and ball game	65
5.4	Toothpick tunnel	67
5.5	Marble can and balance stool	69
5.6	Hole in one game	69
5.7	Zoom ball	69
A.1	Balance board	89
A.2	One-legged balance stool	90
A.3	Finger chart	91

Tables

4.1	Functional vision screening tests	43
4.2	Professionals involved in assessment of visual perception problems	50
4.3	Tests commonly used to evaluate visual perception in children	52
4.4	Understanding test scores	56

INTRODUCTION

Importance of vision to learning and development and the purpose of the book

Vision is commonly described as a child's unique window to the world. More than any other sense, the gift of sight exposes a child to a multitude of experiences that are critical in shaping his or her learning and behavior. Vision is a dynamic process that is far more complex than just being able to see clearly when looking at a stationary object, such as an eye chart. Vision involves looking at multiple stimuli that are constantly changing in time and space, and then being able to interpret the meaning and importance of those stimuli. In order for vision to provide the child with meaningful information, the eyes and their related structures must see clearly, they must move and adjust focus on targets that move in space so that lighting and background are constantly changing, they must attend to relevant detail and ignore irrelevant detail, and they must transmit that information to the brain without distortion. Once this visual information reaches the brain, the brain must interpret or make sense of the information, a process referred to by several different terms, including visual perception, visual information processing, and visual cognition. For the purposes of this book, the term visual perception will be used to refer to the brain's interpretation of visual input. The quality of a child's vision and visual perception affects all aspects of a child's physical, intellectual, emotional, and social growth.

Much has been written about the impact of blindness or serious vision difficulties in children, and how to help these children to learn optimally in a world that deprives them of critical sensory experiences. Less has been written about children who see clearly, but have more subtle vision difficulties that impact their learning and behavior. This is the primary focus of this book. Experts suggest that as many as one in four school-aged children have some degree of vision disorder that impacts their learning. This may seem like a high number until one considers the impact that changing culture has had on human activities. Before the age of computers and standards-based educational outcomes, children spent far more time outdoors, where they used their eyes for a variety of tasks, many of which involved distant viewing and watching moving targets. These days, children spend large amounts of time reading, watching television, playing video games, and working on computers, all of which are more sedentary activities that are less challenging visually because they do not require the eyes to shift frequently from near to far vision. Because vision skills require practice in order to develop, the large amount of time that today's children spend on close visual work can result in strain to the eyes, and may contribute to delays in the development of mature visual skills.

Vision problems are frequently associated with a variety of developmental disabilities. They are very common in children with autism, who often display such behaviors as avoiding eye contact, staring at lights or spinning objects, looking at things from the side of their eyes, and avoiding direct visual attention to their hands during fine motor activities. Many children with autism are over-sensitive to touch or to visual stimulation, and avoid contact with these experiences. Their attention is more focused on the basic body senses related to mental alertness, body position and movement, and touch. Until they learn to process information from these senses in an automatic manner, it is hard for them to attend closely to visual information. Once they are engaged to focus attentively on visual stimuli, they may ignore peripheral vision and remain fixated on the irrelevant details of a task for excessive periods of time. As a result, they often fail to proceed through the typical developmental patterns of visual development, and may have difficulty learning how to use their two eyes together in a coordinated manner, and to remember and make sense of visual information that is critical to learning.

Vision problems are also common in children with attention deficit hyperactivity disorders (AD/HD) and specific learning disabilities, including dyslexia and non-verbal learning disability. Problems with reversals when reading or writing, difficulty learning left from right, poor spatial organization, and poor visual memory, are among the perceptual difficulties that have been well documented in these populations. Problems with efficient use of vision, especially with using the two eyes together (binocular vision) to shift focus onto near point targets, is also a common occurrence among these children. In fact, some experts believe that some children who have been diagnosed with AD/HD are actually misdiagnosed, and that their apparent inattention is really a physical problem with maintaining close visual focus, especially at near point.

Parents and teachers may wonder why these problems go unrecognized in so many children. Unfortunately, as will be seen in later sections of this book, symptoms of vision difficulty can be subtle, and may also fluctuate over time, so they may not be observed at the time of routine vision screenings that are performed in the pediatrician's office or in schools. Also, many children with vision problems fail to complain about blurred or double vision, headaches, or eyestrain because they do not recognize these symptoms as problems. For many children with vision problems, this is the way their eyes have always worked, so they do not realize that other children may actually see things differently.

This book has been designed for parents, teachers, and others who work with children who have developmental delays in learning and behavior, autism spectrum disorders, mild neurologic disorders, or other conditions that may result in poor functional vision or visual perception. The intent is to guide readers to understand how to recognize and screen for subtle problems, understand the options that are available for seeking professional help, learn strategies for coping with problems at home and in the classroom, and identify additional resources for learning more about these issues. The book offers an emphasis on understanding how children may benefit from intervention designed to improve their functional vision and perceptual skills. These interventions are most typically provided by eye doctors (optometrists) who specialize in these disorders, and by occupational therapists, but may also be supported by teachers and other professionals who work with children with special needs. Because vision is, perhaps, the most important sense that a child uses for learning, visual therapy intervention can have a profound effect on overall learning. Changing the way that the visual system functions can, in fact, change the way that the brain is able to process information for learning. It is important to understand that the interventions described in this book cannot, by themselves, alleviate the learning and behavior problems associated with autism, AD/HD, and other learning disabilities. They are not designed to be used as a substitute for medical interventions and special education services. However, vision and perceptual training may be extremely helpful when used as an adjunct to support more traditional medical and educational interventions for these children.

Chapter 1

ANATOMY AND STRUCTURE
OF THE VISUAL SYSTEM

Although it is beyond the scope of this book to provide a comprehensive technical description of the visual system, it is important to have at least a basic understanding of the structures involved and their relationship to perception and to learning. Structurally, the visual system can be thought of as having three distinct parts: 1. the organs of sensation, which are the eyes; 2. the optic nerves, which transmit visual images from the eye and transport it to the brain; and 3. the visual cortex, which is the part of the brain responsible for interpreting information received via the optic nerves. Problems occurring in any part of the visual system can impact the child's perception, and must be considered when selecting appropriate intervention strategies. These three parts of the visual system are interdependent, so that problems in one area can impact another. Clearly, if there is damage to the eyeball that prevents it from taking in an accurate picture, or if the optic nerves fail to transmit images correctly, the brain will not have the information it needs to accurately interpret the picture. Similarly, if the brain receives an accurate picture but does not know how to make sense of the picture because of cognitive or perceptual interferences, the child may not learn what types of visual information he or she needs to pay attention to, and may lose the ability to attend to relevant visual details needed for learning. For this reason, it is important to consider all aspects of vision when attempting to understand a child's visual perceptual skills.

The eye and extraocular muscles

Every sensory system in the human body begins with a peripheral, or distant, organ of sensation. The eye is the peripheral organ for sight, just as the nose is the organ for smell, the skin is the organ for touch, the ear is the organ for hearing, and the tongue is the organ for taste. Figure 1.1 presents a simplified illustration of the structure of the eye.

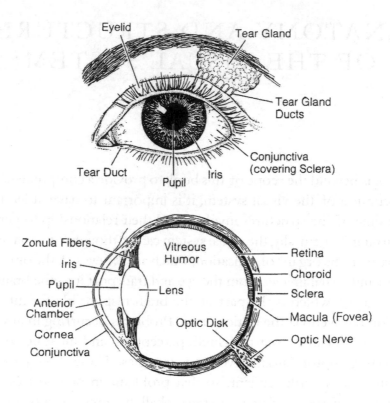

Figure 1.1: Structure of the eye. Reproduced from Miller, Menacker and Batshaw (2002), p.166 with permission from Mark L. Batshaw.

In many ways, the eye functions like a camera. It contains a convex lens system that helps to aim and focus the picture, a variable opening system that allows light to enter, and a structure that records the picture in much the same way as a camera's film. The eyelid helps to keep the eye moist and provides some protection from injury or foreign objects. On the inside of the eyelids lies a thin layer of tissue that contains many tiny blood vessels, called the conjunctiva. Many people are familiar with conjunctivitis, which is an inflammation of this lining due to a viral or bacterial infection, allergy, or other source of irritation. This conjunctival tissue covers most of the white part of the eyeball, which is called the sclera. At the very front of the sclera, conjunctival tissue is replaced by the cornea, which is a transparent structure responsible for allowing light to enter the eye. The cornea covers the iris, which is the colored portion of the eye. The function of the iris is to adjust the amount of light entering the eye by opening and closing its central opening. This central opening is known as the pupil, which is the dark spot in the center of the eyeball. The process of the iris opening and closing to allow light to enter the eye is what makes a person's pupils appear smaller or larger under different conditions. The pupil appears larger under dark conditions, because it is in an open position to allow as much light as possible to enter the eye. Under bright light conditions, the pupil constricts and becomes smaller. When light passes through the cornea, it projects through the lens, which lies directly behind the pupil. The lens further focuses light for projection onto the retina, which is a thin layer of tissue lying in the innermost part of the eye. The retina records the images it receives in an upside down and reversed format, and then transmits the image over the optic nerves to the brain.

The retina contains two types of receptors that change light into nerve impulses for transmission to the brain: the rods and the cones. The cones are concentrated in a small area of the retina called the fovea, or macula, and are the only receptors capable of perceiving color. The cones are responsible for central vision, needed for appreciating fine detail in visual images. Whenever a person needs to have precise vision of a moving target, the eye moves in an effort to keep the image directly focused on the macular portion of the retina. The rods, on the other hand, are scattered throughout the retina, and are responsible for peripheral vision.

Six muscles, called the extraocular muscles, attach to each eye and allow the eye to move in all directions in order to take in visual information from a large field as well as from moving targets. They also ensure that the eyes work together in a well-coordinated fashion, a process known as binocular (two-eyed) vision. Weakness or misalignment of any of these muscles makes it difficult for the eyes to work together in a coordinated manner, and can impact vision significantly. Poor binocular vision can lead to such problems as crossed eyes, double vision, and other problems, which will be discussed further in Chapter 3.

Accommodation describes the process used by the eye to project images clearly onto the retina. Attached to the lens are a number of small muscles, called ciliary muscles. These muscles serve to change the shape of the lens to

allow the eye to focus on objects close up or far away. The ability to accommodate vision to changes in distance is at its best in early childhood and gradually
declines with age. This is why many adults need glasses for reading as they get
older. Their eyes have lost the flexibility to accommodate to view objects at a
close range. Figure 1.2 illustrates the process of accommodation.

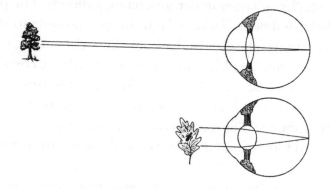

Figure 1.2: Process of accommodation. The lens changes its shape to focus on a near or far object.
Reproduced from Miller, Menacker and Batshaw (2002), p.172 with permission from Mark L. Batshaw.

The optic pathways

Each eye contains one optic nerve that projects from behind the retina on its
way to the brain. Just before the optic nerves enter the brain, some of the fibers
from each nerve cross over to the other side in a structure known as the optic
chiasm, illustrated in Figure 1.3. Each optic nerve now contains some fibers
projecting images from the right eye, and some fibers projecting images from
the left eye, as they continue their pathway towards the brain. As the two optic
nerves reach the brain, they finally each project their images onto one of the
hemispheres of the brain, in the area known as the visual cortex located in the
occipital lobe of the brain. Here, visual information is decoded and sent to the
temporal and parietal lobes of the brain, where perceptual interpretation of the
information takes place.

   In this way, each eye is able to send information to both the right and left
sides of the brain. That is why, if someone loses sight in one eye, the brain con-
tinues to receive a whole picture, although some aspects of vision controlled by

binocular eye movements, especially depth perception, may be impacted. However, this also means that damage to either optic nerve can cause visual disturbances to each hemisphere of the brain, which may result in a loss of some part of the child's field of vision. Problems affecting the optic pathways are not common among children with AD/HD, autism, or learning disabilities, but may be found in some children who have had injuries or illnesses causing brain damage.

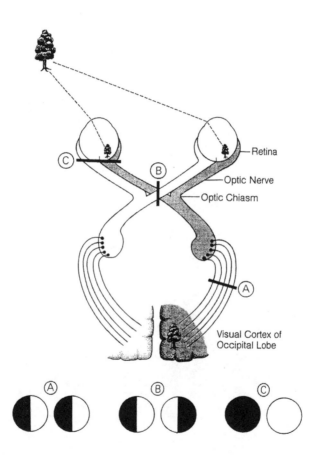

Figure 1.3: Visual pathways. One nerve emerges from behind each eye. A portion of the fibers from each nerve cross at the optic chiasm. An abnormality at various points along the route (upper figure) will lead to different patterns of visual loss (shown as black areas in the lower figures). These are illustrated: A) damage to the cortical pathway; B) damage to the optic chiasm; C) damage to the retina. Reproduced from Miller, Menacker and Batshaw (2002), p.176 with permission from Mark L. Batshaw.

Chapter 2

THE EARLY DEVELOPMENT
OF VISUAL SKILLS

Vision plays a major role in helping the young child to develop cognitive, motor and social skills. As early as six months before birth, the eyes begin preparing for their role, practicing the muscular movements that will allow the eyes to focus on their world after birth. The visual system is anatomically mature at birth. However, the newborn infant does not see things in the same way as an older child or adult, because the visual system must proceed through tremendous developmental maturation as the child experiences and learns from visual input. Vision plays a critical role in all aspects of development, and children born without vision demonstrate characteristic delays impacting motor skills, concept formation, language, and social skills. By the time a child enters school, as much as 75% of classroom teaching uses visual media as a primary instructional tool. Even when learning language, children need visual references and models to understand the meaning and contexts of the words used for teaching.

Visual skills in the first year of life

At birth, the infant recognizes patterns of light and dark, and has reflexive closing of the eyes to bright light. At this early age, the infant's brain responds to any stimulus within its field of vision. However, the eyes can only focus clearly on objects about 8–12 inches away, and the infant is most attracted to objects within this range. Because this is approximately the distance between the infant's eyes and a caregiver's eyes when holding the baby, this mechanism sets the tone for developing the critical eye contact necessary for bonding between infant and caregiver. By about two-and-a-half months of age, the infant will smile in response to making eye contact with a caregiver. The newborn prefers to look at the human face as opposed to other visual stimuli, and this is gradually replaced by interest in black and white designs that are large and that contain clear boundaries, especially with horizontal and vertical markings. At this early age, the infant is more attracted to the edges or boundaries of visual patterns than with the internal portions of a pattern.

Gradually, by about three to four months of age, the infant begins to show interest in all parts of a pattern, and can track visual targets as they move sideways or up and down. At this time, the infant also develops the ability to use the two eyes together (binocular control) to adjust visual focus as objects are moved closer or farther away, a process known as convergence (moving eyes inward towards the nose to look at something close up) and divergence (moving eyes outward to look at objects far away). The development of these movements is the precursor for eye hand coordination, so that by three to four months of age, the infant begins to reach purposefully towards objects. By four months of age, the baby can also see the full range of colors.

As the baby begins to see and to manipulate objects within reach, visual input becomes closely associated with the tactile input to develop an inner language of basic concepts, such as hardness/softness, heavy/light, and round/square. The infant develops an awareness of these basic concepts long before he or she has the language to express an understanding of these concepts. This is the beginning of early visual perceptual development, especially the perception of form, shape, color, size, and other simple attributes.

Between five to seven months of age, the infant's ability to use coordinated binocular eye movements greatly increases. This allows the infant to better judge the location of things in space, and provides motivation to move around and to seek contact with more distant objects. Thus begins the development of such perceptual skills as depth perception and understanding the spatial relationship of objects, which underlies the development of gross and fine motor skills as the infant moves within the environment and contacts objects based on perceptual judgement of their location. At first, the infant must move his or her head or trunk to help aim the eyes towards a desired target, but gradually, eye movement becomes independent of head and trunk movement. Eye movement independent of head and trunk movement does not truly develop until the infant has mature walking and locomotor skills. By about six months of age, the infant usually uses both eyes together when looking at objects.

Because this gives an element of depth to the visual image, infants at this age become more interested in looking at three-dimensional than two-dimensional objects.

Gradually, the infant begins to understand that an object can be viewed from a number of angles, or used in different ways, and still be the same object. He or she learns to recognize familiar objects for what they are, even if partially hidden from view, such as a bottle hidden under a blanket with only the nipple protruding. Objects take on a life of their own, appearing more 'real' to the infant than when viewed as a two-dimensional image, and are missed when they are out of view (the beginning of simple visual memory for form or shape). The infant begins to understand similarities in shape and form, and can begin to place simple shapes in holes.

Other perceptual skills are also emerging at this time, especially form constancy (the ability to recognize an object even if it looks a little different than the way it usually looks) and figure–ground separation (the ability to recognize relevant details even when there are distracting visual elements nearby). These skills develop and start to work in concert with one another, enhancing the infant's understanding of his or her world. At approximately 12 months of age, the infant understands these perceptual concepts well enough to start to use imagery in the form of imitating simple movements or patterns. This ability to imitate represents continued development of visual memory and visual sequencing memory skills. The ability to use imagery is tremendously important in the development of language and cognitive skills. At this age, most infants have also developed visual skills to the extent that they have normal or near-normal visual acuity (the ability to focus clearly on visual targets).

Toddlers and preschoolers

By the time the child is 18 months of age, he or she has much more physical control of the body as needed to negotiate the environment. This is a period of great physical energy and physical exploration of the child's world. The child demonstrates an almost insatiable desire to explore what he or she sees, but has enough physical control of the body that the eyes do not need to guide and direct every movement. For example, the eyes can remain focused on a distant target or destination during walking. The child has enough sense of body awareness that he or she can walk without having to watch their feet during every step. The child gradually begins to be able to focus on objects farther and farther away. Depth perception reaches 4 to 10 feet by 18 months, 10 to 16 feet by 3 years, 16 to 20 feet by 4 years, and 20 feet or greater by the time the child enters kindergarten. Peripheral vision also increases greatly during the pre-school years, so the child becomes more aware of visual images outside of his or her direct line of vision. These developing skills further increase the child's interest in language to describe the relationship of objects to one another. Concepts such as next to, behind, close or far become integrated into the child's use of language to describe simple spatial relationships.

Fine motor skills also develop tremendously during the preschool years, and there is an increased interest in activities that involve using the hands to build, draw, cut, and paste. Eye and hand movements become intimately inte-grated, but the eyes do not need to guide every movement because the child develops a visual image combined with motor memory of the movements needed to complete familiar tasks.

Increased maturity of visual skills also play an important role in the devel-opment of social skills during this period. As the child can focus and attend visually to more distant and peripheral targets, and as he or she becomes more sensitive to recognizing the subtleties of visual images, the child learns to reach out to negotiate social interactions with others using non-verbal communica-tion methods. The eyes help the child to recognize subtle body language meant as an invitation to engage with others, such as when to initiate conversation or to join in play. As the child interprets facial expression, hand gestures, and other forms of body language, these visual cues guide the way in which the child initi-ates and maintains social relationships with others. In these ways, vision plays a contributory role in all aspects of the child's participation in his or her world.

Chapter 3

DO YOU SEE WHAT I SEE?
PROBLEMS WITH VISUAL SKILLS

There are many different types of vision problems that may occur in children. Some are caused by physical abnormalities to the eyes or its related structures. These may be present at birth or caused by injury or illness, and are referred to as *structural* vision problems. Other vision difficulties are caused by problems that affect the efficiency of the visual system. These are referred to as *functional* vision problems. Finally, even if the visual system is physically intact and works efficiently, visual information must be interpreted correctly by the brain. Problems with this interpretation are called *visual perception* problems. This chapter will describe some of the more common vision problems that children may have.

Structural vision problems

Physical impairments of the eyes, the optic nerves, or the parts of the brain that process visual information can cause vision problems ranging from mild to severe. The majority of children described as having significant vision impairment are diagnosed with the problem at or shortly after birth, while less than a quarter are the result of a condition acquired later in life. Often, these impairments are not able to be corrected through medical intervention, and result in lifelong challenges to learning. Functional and perceptual vision problems usually co-exist with structural impairments. Although this type of vision problem is not the primary focus of this book, some of the more common structural vision problems identified in children are described below:

- *Anophthalmia* refers to congenital absence of the eyeball, resulting in total blindness from birth.

- *Albinism* is a genetic condition that results in a partial or total lack of pigment in the hair, skin, and eyes. Many children with albinism are excessively sensitive to bright light because their irises function inefficiently. The absence of pigment may also affect the retina, causing vision impairment that is not always correctable through lenses.

- *Color blindness* is a genetic condition caused by absence of one or more of the three types of cone cells. It occurs in 5% to 8% of males, and in less than 1% of females. It is extremely rare for an individual to have no color vision, that is, to see everything in black and white. Most commonly, there is limited perceptual sensitivity to red-green or to yellow-blue.

- *Congenital cataracts* are an opacity or cloudiness of the lens that is present before birth, most commonly as a result of a disturbance to the developing eye during the mother's pregnancy. Cataracts prevent light from reaching the retina, and are treated by surgically removing the lens. With the lens removed, the eye is no longer able to focus, so the child must use glasses, contact lenses, or have a surgically implanted artificial lens to see. Many children with congenital cataracts have severely impaired vision even with corrective lenses.

- *Congenital glaucoma* refers to increased fluid pressure within the eye, and is usually related to a genetic condition. If left untreated, the pressure gradually builds, exerting pressure on the blood vessels of the retina, and potentially leading to blindness.

- *Cortical blindness* occurs when the areas of the brain that process visual information are congenitally absent, or are damaged as a result of neurological infection, injury, hydrocephalus, or a lack of oxygen to the brain. This type of vision impairment is almost always associated with other developmentally disabling conditions. Although some recovery often occurs, many children with this condition remain severely visually impaired.

- *Hemianopsia* refers to loss of one half of the visual field, which may occur in one or both eyes, caused by damage to one or more parts of the visual pathways. The various types of field loss are illustrated in Figure 1.3.

- *Leber's amaurosis* is a congenital disorder, more common in boys than girls, that results in severe, sudden vision loss in early infancy. Although peripheral vision may return, the condition is associated with a loss of central vision.

- *Macular degeneration* refers to the loss of central vision caused by congenital malformation or disease affecting the macula. The macula is the small, circular area near the center of the retina that contains cones and is responsible for central vision and vision of fine detail. Children with this condition usually have normal peripheral vision, and can move around their environment without significant difficulty, but have significant difficulty using vision to read or process other visual information important to the learning process.

- *Optic nerve atrophy* occurs when some or all of the fibers in the optic nerve are damaged as a result of injury, infection, tumor, lack of oxygen, or maldevelopment of the nervous system. This causes permanent loss of function of the optic nerve, and is the most common eye abnormality among children with severe vision impairment.

- *Optic nerve hypoplasia* occurs when the optic nerves fail to develop fully, and remain smaller than normal. Children with this condition often have other brain abnormalities that further impact their development.

- *Retinopathy of prematurity* is a vision impairment that is very common in low birthweight, premature infants. It is the result of an overgrowth of retinal tissue due to underdeveloped blood vessels in that portion of the eye. The excess retinal tissue can cause the retina to detach, and may cause varying degrees of vision impairment.

- *Retinitis pigmentosa* is a hereditary condition of the retina that results from progressive degeneration of the rods. Children with this disorder become progressively less able to adapt to lower levels of light, and gradually lose their peripheral vision, resulting in tunnel vision.

Functional vision impairments

Functional vision impairments are the result of problems that cause the eyes to function inefficiently. They may be thought of as falling into one of two sub-categories: 1. *refractive errors* (problems with how light is reflected off the retina) and 2. *visual efficiency disorders* (problems with using smooth, well-coordinated muscle control to allow the eyes to gather necessary visual information).

Visual acuity is only one aspect of vision, but perhaps the best understood. It refers to how clearly someone can see a stationary object under highly controlled conditions. Distance vision refers to how clearly someone can see a target placed 20 feet away, and is usually tested using a Snellen Chart (recognizing letters that become progressively smaller) or other similar methods that have been designed for children who do not yet know their letters. Normal vision is 20/20, meaning that the individual sees objects 20 feet away as clearly as normal people. Visual acuity of 20/100 means that an individual can see clearly at 20 feet what normal people can see clearly from 100 feet away. Legal blindness occurs when a person's vision in their better eye is less than 20/200 using glasses, or when the field of vision is restricted to an angle of 20° or less. Many people are surprised to learn that people who have been diagnosed with legal blindness may, in fact, have very useful remaining vision.

Refractive errors

Myopia, or nearsightedness, occurs when the light rays entering the eye are focused in front of the retina, causing blurred vision. This occurs either because the eye shape is elongated, or the refractive mechanism of the eye is too strong. Children with myopia can see objects clearly when they are close up, but have difficulty seeing objects clearly at a distance. Children with uncorrected myopia may squint when looking at things far away, because the squinting creates a temporary pinhole effect that improves clarity. Glasses with concave lenses help to refocus the image onto the fovea. Functionally, children with myopia may prefer sedentary activities that involve the use of close vision, such as reading or drawing, over more active, physical exploration of the environment. This may explain, at least in part, the incorrect stereotype that nearsighted children are smarter than other children.

Hyperopia, or farsightedness, occurs when light rays focus behind the retina, and cause the individual to have difficulty focusing on objects that are close to the eyes. This is by far the most common refractive error among children. It occurs when the eye shape is too spherical, or when the refracting mechanism is too weak. Hyperopia differs from myopia in that the individual may be able to compensate for the problem by voluntarily contracting the ciliary muscles of the eye, thus changing the shape of the lens. In this way, light is reflected closer to the retina and clarity of vision improves. Children with mild hyperopia have excellent acuity and may require no correction through glasses. However, more significant degrees of hyperopia can lead to problems caused by the constant muscular effort required to maintain visual focus, and can result in blurred vision, eyestrain, tearing, and discomfort during visual tasks. Glasses with convex lenses may be used to correct this problem.

Astigmatism is another type of refractive disorder, and occurs when the eye is shaped more like an American football. This causes the light entering the eye to focus on two different points, and can cause blurring of vision at both

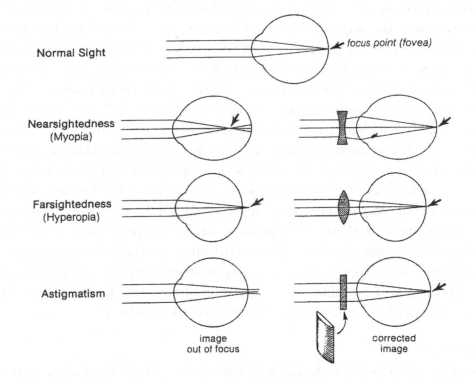

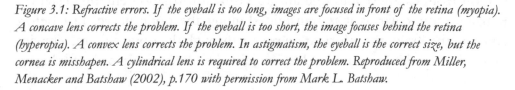

Figure 3.1: Refractive errors. If the eyeball is too long, images are focused in front of the retina (myopia). A concave lens corrects the problem. If the eyeball is too short, the image focuses behind the retina (hyperopia). A convex lens corrects the problem. In astigmatism, the eyeball is the correct size, but the cornea is misshapen. A cylindrical lens is required to correct the problem. Reproduced from Miller, Menacker and Batshaw (2002), p.170 with permission from Mark L. Batshaw.

near and far points. Glasses with a cylindrically shaped lens can correct this problem. Children with hyperopia or astigmatism may complain of headaches, tearing, or discomfort during reading or other tasks requiring close visual scrutiny, which may lead to avoidance of these activities. Figure 3.1 illustrates the various types of refractive errors in children, and how lenses are used to correct the problem.

Visual efficiency disorders

Visual efficiency disorders refer to problems with eye muscle control that prevent an individual from comfortably gathering visual information as needed for function. These problems can be classified as problems with 1. *accommodation*; 2. *binocular vision*; and 3. *ocular motility*.

ACCOMMODATION

Accommodation is the ability to contract the ciliary muscles surrounding the lens to change the shape of the lens. This allows the individual to change the focus of the eye to see things closer or farther away. The ability to accommodate is related to age. Newborns are unable to accommodate, and can focus only on objects fairly close to their eyes. By approximately six months of age, however, children can be expected to accommodate as well as young adults. Young children typically have greater accommodative ability than older adults, who gradually lose the muscular elasticity needed for accommodation, a condition known as *presbyopia*. This is the reason why most adults must eventually resort to using reading glasses when doing close visual work. Accommodative disorders exist when either 1. accommodation is less than expected; 2. accommodation speed is slower than average; or 3. accommodation cannot be sustained over time. Accommodative difficulties generally create functional problems when using the eyes for reading or other near tasks. Symptoms may include blurred vision, headaches, eyestrain, a sensation of pulling around the eyes, excessive fatigue, reading problems, and task avoidance.

BINOCULAR VISION

Binocular vision refers to the ability of the visual system to combine the information from each eye into one image. Visual information entering each eye remains monocular as it is transmitted along the optic nerve. Just before entering the brain, the information passes through the optic chiasm, allowing binocular visual information to be transmitted to the brain. In order for binoc-

ular vision to occur, the information gathered by each eye must be equal in clarity and size. Problems with alignment of the eyes, or with unequal refractive errors, can contribute to problems with binocular vision. *Diplopia*, or double vision, is the primary symptom of poor binocular vision.

Misalignment of the eyes is known as *strabismus*. It may be caused by a variety of factors, including abnormal focusing ability, a weakness in the eye muscles, a disorder in one of the nerves that controls eye muscles, or in the part of the brain that controls eye movements. Six pairs of muscles, known as *extraocular muscles*, surround the eyes and control their movement as gaze is directed towards a visual target. As illustrated in Figure 3.2, when these muscles are imbalanced, the child's eye may turn in (*esotropia*), turn out (*exotropia*), or turn upwards (*hypertropia*).

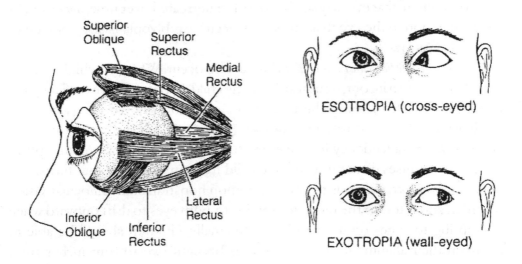

Figure 3.2: The eye muscles. Six muscles move the eyeball. A weakness of one of these muscles causes strabismus. In esotropia, the eyeball turns in, whereas in exotropia, the eyeball turns out. Reproduced from Miller, Menacker and Batshaw (2002), p.178 with permission from Mark L. Batshaw.

When the eyes are misaligned, each eye is focused on a different visual image, and therefore sends a different picture to the brain, which interprets the information as double vision. Strabismus may be present all of the time, or may be intermittent, meaning that the child has adequate binocular vision at least some of the time.

Because the brain finds double vision to be uncomfortable to interpret, it may attempt to eliminate the problem through one of two mechanisms: 1. using muscular effort to re-align the weaker eye, or 2. allowing the brain to ignore or "turn off" one of the double images, an adaptation that is called *suppression*. Both of these mechanisms are easier to apply when the child is younger than age six or when the strabismus is intermittent. Therefore, mild or intermittent strabismus may go unnoticed during routine eye examinations. Even when children are able to use muscular effort to re-align their eyes, a number of problems may occur as a result of the effort. Headaches, eyestrain, blurred vision, intermittent double vision, and difficulty sustaining visual attention are common complaints in these children. When young children suppress one of a double image, that eye no longer receives visual stimulation, and the visual development of that eye may be halted. If left untreated over time, *amblyopia*, or a loss of vision in the eye that turns, may occur. Amblyopia is also sometimes referred to as lazy eye.

Nonstrabismic binocular vision disorders can also occur. When the child's eye has a tendency to turn in, out, or upward, but the child can control the tendency, the condition is called *phoria*. The three most common phorias are *esophoria* (a tendency for the eye to turn in), *exophoria* (a tendency for the eye to turn out), and *hyperphoria* (a tendency for the eye to turn upward). Phoria becomes problematic if it causes discomfort for the child to control the eye that turns.

Convergence insufficiency is the most common nonstrabismic binocular vision disorder, and refers to the tendency for one or both eyes to drift outward when attempting to focus on a near object. Normally, children should be able to maintain their alignment until an object is brought two to four inches from their eyes, at which point double vision occurs.

OCULAR MOTILITY DISORDERS

Ocular motility disorders include problems with visual fixation, visual tracking or scanning, and saccades. Saccades are rapid eye movements that redirect the line of sight so that the point of interest stimulates the fovea. Ocular motility skills are particularly important during reading, which requires rapid and skillful movement of the eyes to maintain focus on the print. Children with ocular motility disorders may have poor attention during reading, frequently lose their place, skip lines, or use excessive head movement to follow the print. They may also demonstrate developmental delays with coloring, drawing, or writing.

Visual perception problems

Visual perception may be thought of as the cognitive component of interpreting visual stimuli, or more simply, understanding what is seen. It involves the ability to mentally manipulate visual information as needed to solve problems and to take action in response to environmental demands. Visual perception is an extremely critical component of a child's learning. Children with problems affecting visual perception have difficulty recognizing, remembering, and organizing visual images as needed to understand the written and pictorial symbols that are used for learning. They often have trouble learning to read, but may also have difficulty understanding the symbols used in learning other subjects involving diagrams, maps, charts, or graphs. Visual perception problems often co-exist with structural or functional vision disorders, but also commonly occur in children without these disorders. Many children with good eyesight who have developmental delays, learning disabilities, or neurological conditions also demonstrate problems with visual perception.

Visual perception involves a number of related abilities that tend to be interdependent upon one another. It is hard to define explicitly one type of perceptual problem from another, and some specialists define problems using different terminology. However, the following terms are frequently used to describe common problems with visual perception:

- *Visual attention* refers to the child's alertness and readiness for active learning using visual stimuli. It requires a conscious effort to concentrate and persist with looking, and to use the muscles of the eyes to efficiently focus on visual stimuli. Visual attention also requires the child to notice visual stimuli that may be peripheral to the task at hand, and to select which stimuli are relevant to attend to, and which can be ignored. Children with problems affecting visual attention may fail to notice relevant details that should guide their learning or behavior, or may become overwhelmed by visual detail that should be ignored.

- *Visual closure* refers to the ability to recognize forms or objects that are missing parts or are incompletely presented. This skill allows the child to quickly recognize an object by mentally completing the visual image or by relating the image to previously stored information. It is this skill that allows the infant to recognize his or her bottle when it is partly hidden under a blanket, or that allows an adult to read quickly by skimming over the words in a passage. Problems with visual closure may contribute to reading or spelling difficulties in children.

- *Visual form constancy* is the ability to recognize that forms and objects remain the same even if they are seen in different environments or have different positions or sizes. This allows the young child to relate to a two-dimensional picture of a familiar object, such as a block or doll, and recognize it for what it represents. It allows the child to recognize that a familiar object, such as a car, seen at a distance is really larger than it appears. It is also the skill that allows an emerging reader to quickly recognize the letter 'A' whether it is in lowercase or uppercase, manuscript or cursive, and in different fonts or forms.

- *Visual discrimination* refers to the ability to recognize the basic features of stimuli, such as shape, size, orientation or color. The ability to sort or match objects by these features reflects the ability to use visual discrimination skills. Some specialists refer to this type of visual perception as *visual form perception*.

- *Visual figure–ground discrimination* allows the child to separate foreground from background visual information in order to attend to the relevant details. It is what allows the child to focus quickly on the most important aspects of the visual image, while retaining an awareness of the relationships of parts to the whole image. Children with problems in this area may have difficulty learning when there are too many words or other images on the pages they must look at. They frequently lose their place when doing visual work.

- *Visual memory* refers to the ability to recall visually presented material. There are different types of visual memory, including immediate recall of information (sometimes called *working memory*), longer-term recall of information, and recall of the exact order of a series of items (called *visual sequential memory*).

- *Visual-motor integration* refers to the ability to integrate visual information with fine motor movement. It is the skill that allows the child to anticipate where to place his or her hand in order to catch a moving ball, or how to move the hand in a precise manner to write a letter or word. This skill implies a dynamic process, where the child is continually adjusting his or her movement based upon the visual feedback that occurs during the course of the movement. Visual-motor integration is a critical component of early childhood learning, which tends to use manipulatives and other "hands on" approaches. It is the skill that underlies learning to cut with scissors, use a pencil, manage clothing fasteners, and manipulate a variety of toys, and classroom tools and materials. Some specialists use the term *eye hand coordination* to describe this type of perceptual skill.

- *Visual-spatial perception* refers to the child's ability to recognize the orientation and position of objects, as well as the orientation of self to the environment. It is what allows the child to recognize left from right, up from down, and top from bottom, and to learn the vocabulary used to describe these relationships. Children with this type of perceptual problem frequently reverse letters, numbers or words. However, it is important to recognize that understanding of spatial relationships develops gradually over the early school years. Reversals are not uncommon in typically developing second graders, who can often recognize that they have made a reversal. Visual-spatial perception also contributes to an awareness of depth perception, and to developing a cognitive "map" of the environment, which helps the child learn to plan how to move around efficiently within his or her environment.

Chapter 4

FINDING PROFESSIONAL HELP
FOR PROBLEMS WITH VISION

Fortunately, the majority of children are born with normal, healthy eyes. Most children with problems involving eye health, structure, or significant vision impairment are easily identified by pediatricians responsible for their care, and are referred for medical treatment and early developmental intervention as needed. Thanks to routine early periodic screening for all children, less serious problems affecting visual acuity (nearsightedness, farsightedness, and astigmatism), as well as serious problems with misalignment of the eyes (strabismus) are usually identified no later than when the child enters kindergarten. However, milder problems with vision are often undetected during routine vision screenings. Not all children with apparently healthy eyes and good acuity are able to use their eyes efficiently, and these children may suffer from functional vision difficulties that impact their perception and participation in daily activities. In fact, some experts contend that as many as 50% of students who experience learning difficulties in school may have some degree of functional vision disorder.

Visual perceptual differences are commonly found in children with autism spectrum disorders and learning disabilities, especially non-verbal learning disorders. Studies have also shown a potential link between attention deficit hyperactivity disorder (AD/HD) and vision difficulties. Symptoms of these milder forms of functional vision disorder can be difficult to notice by an untrained observer, especially since they may fluctuate over time. Often, children who have these problems do not complain to parents about blurred or double vision, eyestrain, or headaches, because they simply do not recognize that these could be signs of a problem. For these reasons, functional vision problems may not be picked up during a routine eye exam that focuses primarily on assessment of acuity and general alignment of the eyes. Therefore, it is extremely important for parents, teachers, and other professionals to learn to recognize the signs and symptoms of functional vision disorders, and to understand how to make a referral to the appropriate professionals for further evaluation of suspected problems. This chapter attempts to educate the reader about screening for potential problems, understanding the processes and terminology used in various types of formal vision assessment, and appreciating the similarities and differences between various vision specialists.

Warning signs of functional vision and perceptual disorders

Symptoms that are suggestive of functional vision disorders may relate to the *appearance* of the eyes, the *behavior* of the child when performing tasks that require close visual attention, or *complaints* made by the child either during or immediately after using the eyes. Symptoms are considered more significant when they persist over time, or when there is a pattern of symptoms that routinely occurs either during or immediately after specific visual activities, such as reading or writing. If a problem is suspected, it is often helpful to consider the presence or absence of symptoms in different settings, as this might offer clues as to the nature of the problem. For example, children who find it hard to use their eyes efficiently for reading may avoid reading at home, and therefore appear relatively symptom-free when observed by family members. However, their symptoms may be more prominent in the school setting, where the student is obliged to participate in sustained reading activities on a daily basis.

The following are symptoms of vision disorder that affect the *appearance* of the eyes. These should generally be brought to the attention of the child's pediatrician before considering any type of specialized vision assessment, because they may require medical intervention.

- Eyes turn in or out. Note that this is fairly common and typical in infants younger than two months, but should not occur in older children. One way to check for this is to turn off the lights, then shine a pinpoint flashlight directly at the bridge of the child's nose when he or she is looking straight at the light, then at a target that is directly behind the adult at some distance away from the child. The light should reflect in the same area of each pupil if the eyes are properly aligned.

- Crusting, swelling, or drooping of the eyelids.

- Redness of eyes or lids (suggests conjunctivitis).

- Persistent tearing.

- Squinting in normal sunlight or under fluorescent lights.

- Frowning or squinting when looking closely at objects.

The following list indicates *behaviors* that may be observed in a child who is experiencing visual difficulties. The presence of one or more of these symptoms combined with poor school achievement suggests the need for formal vision assessment:

- Frequent squinting or rubbing of the eyes.

- Disinterest in or avoidance of activities that require close visual attention.

- General clumsiness, frequently bumps into or drops things, poor judgment as to the distance of objects, difficulty throwing at a target or catching a ball.

- Poor handwriting, difficulty learning correct letter formations, frequent erasures, uneven spacing, difficulty using margins.

- Reversals of letters, numbers, or words. This is a normal part of development that usually resolves by the end of second grade. Persistent confusion with reversals after second grade, or inability to recognize and correct reversals in a younger student, is cause for concern.

- Difficulty copying from the board, or general difficulty with the writing process. Omits letters from words and words from sentences, poor organization of ideas, can spell phonetically but has poor immediate recall of the spelling of basic sight words.

- Poor reading comprehension despite good vocabulary and spoken language skills.

- Difficulty with higher level math concepts (e.g., time, money, carrying, graphs, etc.).

- Daydreaming, or difficulty concentrating or attending, especially during reading or other activities requiring visual attention.

- Tilting the head, or covering or closing one eye during reading.

- Moving the head to follow a line of print, instead of moving the eyes independently of the head.

- Persistently holding books or worksheets in an unusual position.

- Difficulty keeping place during reading—skipping lines or words.

Children with learning or achievement problems may have *complaints* of physical or visual discomfort that may suggest an underlying vision deficit. This is highly variable, however, as often children have experienced the symptoms for as long as they can remember, and do not recognize the symptom as anything irregular. The following list suggests symptoms that may require formal vision assessment:

- Frequent headaches during or following reading.

- Eyes ache or burn.

- Blurred or double vision when using the eyes.

- Difficulty seeing the whiteboard, charts, or other visual targets at a distance.

- Words disappear or jump about during reading.

- Nausea or dizziness during or immediately following reading.

- Excessive fatigue at the end of the school day.

Selecting a vision specialist

When problems with functional vision or cognitive visual perception are suspected, it is appropriate to seek further assessment by someone with specialized training and experience in these problems. However, because there are many different types of professionals who may address visual difficulties, parents and teachers are often confused as to where to begin searching for help. Because cognitive aspects of visual perception are dependent upon good visual efficiency, it is probably a good idea to begin by ruling out functional vision deficits (such as problems with oculomotor control, eye teaming, and binocular control) before or in combination with assessment of cognitive perceptual skills (such as visual memory, spatial perception, and figure–ground separation).

For children with identified developmental disabilities, including autism, AD/HD, learning disabilities, or other diagnoses that significantly impact development and learning, a good place to start is with the nurse or occupational therapist who has regular contact with the child. Often, these professionals have the skills needed to screen for functional vision deficits and to assist in making a referral to the appropriate eye specialist if needed. Clinical assessment of visual skills should minimally consist of the following procedures:

- *Near vision acuity*. Using a Snellen Chart, rotating E chart, or other method suitable for children who do not yet recognize letters. Acuity of 20/40 or poorer should indicate a need for referral.

- *Convergence insufficiency*. Have the child focus on a small target (popsicle stick with sticker, or pencil with topper) from a distance of approximately 15 inches. As the target is slowly brought towards the nose, the two eyes should remain on the target, slowly moving inwards. Convergence is broken when the child reports double vision, or when the two eyes no longer remain focused on the target. This should occur at two to four inches from the nose.

- *Ocular tracking*. Using a small target held approximately 12 inches from the eyes, slowly move the target horizontally and vertically, then to all positions using a "figure eight" pattern. Observe the eyes for signs of jerkiness or incoordination, or for difficulty when crossing the midline of the body during tracking.

- *Saccades*. Hold two different targets in front of the child's shoulders from a distance of approximately 12 inches. Have the child shift focus from one target to the other without moving his or her head. Each time the child focuses on one target, move the other target up or down vertically before asking the child to shift focus. Observe the eyes for accuracy and speed of focus, or for difficulty moving the eyes independently of the head.

- *Alignment*. Seated in a dark room, shine a pinpoint flashlight directly at the bridge of the child's nose when he or she is looking straight at the light, then at a target that is directly behind the adult at some distance away from the child. The light should reflect in the same area of each pupil if the eyes are properly aligned.

- *Cover test for strabismus.* Have the child focus on a distant target with both eyes. While the child is focusing, cover one eye. If the uncovered eye moves, it was not focusing on the target, suggesting the presence of strabismus. Repeat for the other eye at distance, then screen each eye when focusing on a near target. This test should be performed slowly, allowing a few seconds between each cover to allow the eyes to relax.

In addition to a clinical assessment of visual acuity, fields of vision, and control of eye muscles, these professionals may use one or more standardized screening tools to determine the need for further referral. Table 4.1 lists examples of screening tests for functional vision in children.

If screening suggests that a specialized eye examination is indicated, it is usually necessary to first contact the child's pediatrician to obtain a referral. It is very important to explain to the pediatrician the exact nature of the concerns, and to make sure that the examination will address all aspects of the child's vision, not just eye health, visual acuity, and alignment. Many insurance companies will require that the child's pediatrician authorize a referral for evaluation by a vision specialist.

There are two kinds of eye doctors that may be recommended by the pediatrician, and each have different educational backgrounds and philosophical approaches to care. *Ophthalmologists* are medical doctors whose training includes a residency in ophthalmology, additional post-graduate training in pediatric ophthalmology ranging from three to eight years after the completion of medical school, and board certification. They use the initials M.D. after their name to indicate their training as a medical doctor. Ophthalmologists are surgeons who specialize in medical and surgical interventions for disorders of the eyes and vision. Problems with eye health or structure are appropriately referred to this type of specialist, as are severe problems with ocular motility. However, it is important to recognize that their approach to treatment of functional vision deficits is usually limited to prescription lenses for refractive errors, and use of patching, prescription eye drops, or surgery to correct muscle imbalance. Most ophthalmologists are not oriented towards the relationship of functional vision to learning, and do not provide specific intervention for these problems.

Optometrists are primary health providers who complete a four-year graduate training program in optometry after completing undergraduate school. They are not trained as general medical doctors, but do specialize in the management

Table 4.1 Functional vision screening tests

Title and description	Source
Disorders of the Visual Perception System This chapter describes comprehensive screening measures for distance and near vision acuity, convergence, horizontal pursuits, ocular fixation, and binocular vision skills.	Bouska, M.J., Kauffman, N. and Marcus, S.E. (1990) "Disorders of the visual perception system." In D. Umphred (Ed.) *Neurological Rehabilitation, Second Edition*, St. Louis: Mosby Yearbook, 522–585
Erhardt Developmental Vision Assessment Measures motor components of vision up to six months of age, which is considered to be the age of visual maturity. Therefore, this test can be used for older children. Measures both reflexive visual patterns and voluntary eye movements including localization, fixation, ocular pursuits and gaze shift.	Erhardt, R.P. (1989) *Erhardt Developmental Vision Assessment, Revised Edition*. Therapy Skill Builders, 555 Academic Court, San Antonio, TX 78204
McDowell Vision Screening Kit Screening test suitable for even very young children or those with severe disabilities. Assesses near point and distance acuity, ocular alignment and motility, color perception, and ocular function.	McDowell, P.M. and McDowell, R.L. (1994) *McDowell Vision Screening Kit*. Western Psychological Services, 12031 Wilshire Boulevard, Los Angeles, CA 90025-1251
NYSOA Vision Battery Easy to use screening test that assesses 16 aspects of functional vision.	Cohen, A., Ritty, M., Lieberman, S. and Stolzber, M. (1986) *NYSOA Vision Battery*. Bernell Corporation, 750 Lincolnway East, P.O. Box 4637, South Bend, IN 46634-4637
Pediatric Clinical Vision Screening for Occupational Therapists Screening test for accommodation, binocular vision, and ocular motility.	Scheiman, M. (1991) *Pediatric Clinical Vision Screening for Occupational Therapists*. Pennsylvania College of Optometry, 8360 Old York Road, Elkins Park, PA 19027-1598
Visual Skills Appraisal Individually administered, norm-referenced test for children five to nine years of age. Measures pursuits, scanning, alignment, locating movements, eye hand coordination, and fixation unity. Subtests scores are converted to a scale that provides cut-off points suggesting the need for further evaluation.	Richards, R.G. (1984) *Visual Skills Appraisal*. Academic Therapy Publications, 20 Commercial Boulevard, Novato, CA 94949-6191

of diseases and disorders of the eyes and the visual system. They tend to use a more holistic approach to the treatment of vision disorders than ophthalmologists, and are more focused or the role that vision plays in the quality of that individual's daily lifestyle. Professionals who have completed training as an optometrist use the initials O.D. after their name. Many optometrists undergo post-graduate education to specialize in some aspect of vision care, such as geriatric care, prescribing contact lenses, or providing assistive devices and aids for people with very limited vision who cannot perform daily living skills independently. A small number of optometrists choose to specialize in children's vision, and complete extensive post-graduate training to practice as specialists in this area.

There are two organizations that offer examinations for optometrists to assess their level of expertise in this area. Optometrists who pass the examination given by the American Academy of Optometry are called Diplomates in Binocular Vision, Perception, and Pediatric Optometry. Optometrists who pass the examination offered by the College of Optometrists in Vision Development (COVD) are called Fellows of the COVD, and use the initials FCOVD after their name. While other optometrists may offer vision therapy as part of their practice, optometrists who have either of these advanced credentials are most likely to have a high level of expertise in providing vision therapy for children.

Some people also use the terms *developmental* or *behavioral optometrist* to describe this type of professional. Besides offering typical assessment of refractive errors, developmental/behavioral optometrists provide specialized vision therapy that may include special lenses, exercises, and other training methods to strengthen visual skills and to reduce visual stress. This type of vision therapy may be thought of as a type of physical therapy for the eyes, and may help to correct such problems as wandering eyes, lazy eyes, poor eye teaming and tracking, visual-motor integration problems, and visual perceptual disorders. The interventions that are recommended by a developmental/behavioral optometrist will be highly individualized to the needs of the child, and may include any of the following:

- prescription glasses
- prisms
- a patch to temporarily occlude one eye
- office-based vision therapy

- home or school programs to support vision development
- recommendations for environmental modifications to support visual efficiency
- low vision aids, such as magnifiers.

Understanding the differences between these types of eye doctors, it is recommended that serious problems with eye health should be referred to an ophthalmologist, and suspected refractive errors be referred to either an ophthalmologist or an optometrist. However, if significant problems with functional vision are suspected, referral to a developmental/behavioral optometrist may be the most prudent choice. Few pediatricians will make a referral to a developmental/behavioral optometrist unless they are presented with a compelling argument for the need. This is due to several reasons. Typically, health insurance covers eye examinations for eye health problems, and may, depending upon the particular insurance, cover examination for refractive errors. The coverage for functional vision examination is much more variable. Also, because a relatively small number of optometrists have completed the necessary training as a specialist in children's vision, they may not be included in a particular insurance company's network of approved providers. Finally, some pediatricians are unaware of the difference between a regular optometrist and one who is specially trained to assess children's functional vision, or may hold a bias against the potential benefits of vision therapy over more traditional medical management. While early research examining the benefits of vision therapy was inconclusive, methods have evolved in recent years, and the benefits of current approaches to vision therapy are now well documented. The American Optometric Association offers a free publication entitled *The Efficacy of Optometric Vision Therapy* that lists multiple references of research studies supporting the use of vision therapy. Some parents who lack insurance coverage or their pediatrician's support for an evaluation by a developmental/behavioral optometrist may choose to pay out of pocket for at least an initial evaluation to better understand their child's difficulties. Even if they are unable to pay for longer-term therapy without the help of insurance, the information from an evaluation can be of enormous benefit to the parents, teachers, and therapists who work with the child on a daily basis. Also, there may be informal interventions and accommodations that can be made for the child following an evaluation. Some of these will be described in the following chapter.

Several organizations offer directories or referral programs to assist in locating a developmental/behavioral optometrist. These are listed below:

Organizations with directories of optometrists offering vision therapy

UNITED STATES

American Academy of Optometry
6110 Executive Boulevard, Suite 506
Rockville, MD 20852
Telephone: (301) 984-1441
Website: www.aaopt.org/

College of Optometrists in Vision Development
243 N. Lindbergh Boulevard, Suite 310
St. Louis, MO 63141
Telephone: (888) 268-3770
Website: www.covd.org/

Optometric Extension Program
1921 E. Carnegie Avenue, Suite 3-L
Santa Ana, CA 92705-5510
Telephone: (949) 250-8070
Website: www.oep.org/

The Optometrists Network
93 Bedford Street, Suite 5D
New York, NY 10014
Website: www.vision3d.com or *http://optometrists.org/*

OUTSIDE OF THE UNITED STATES

American Academy of Optometry (British Chapter)
2 Doric Place
Woodbridge, Suffolk IP12 1BT, UK
Telephone: (0)1394 380139
Website: www.academy.org.uk/

Australasian College of Behavioral Optometrists
Harmony Vision Center
17 Christine Avenue
Burleigh Waters, Queensland, Australia 4220
Telephone: (07) 5520 5900
Website: www.acbo.org.au/

British Association of Behavioural Optometrists
c/o Aquila Optometrists
72 High Street
Billericay, Essex CM12 9BS UK
Telephone: (0)1277 624916
Email: aquila72@aol.com

Canadian Association of Optometrists
234 Argyle Avenue
Ottawa, Ontario
Canada K2P 1B9
Telephone: (888) 263-4676
Website: www.opto.ca/en/public/

Optometrists Association Australia
P.O. Box 185
Carlton, South Victoria, Australia 3053
Telephone: (03) 9663 6833
Website: www.optometrists.asn.au/

Another option is to contact local colleges or universities that offer programs in optometric training to ask for their advice about a referral. The following list offers questions to ask an eye doctor prior to making an appointment. This will help to ensure that the doctor has the appropriate training and approach to visual assessment.

- Do you have experience working with children who have developmental and learning disabilities?
- Do you test accommodative amplitude and facility?
- Do you evaluate fusional vergence amplitude and facility?
- Do you evaluate visual information processing skills?
- Do you offer vision therapy services?

- Will you train me how to help my child at home, under your supervision?

- Will you send a report to my child's teacher and other professionals that includes recommendations for helping him or her at school?

Regardless of the type of specialist who provides an eye examination, parents should request that a report be shared both with parents and with school personnel. Often, medical reports can include unfamiliar language that is difficult for the untrained person to understand. Hopefully, the glossary included in this book will help to define some of the terminology that might be included in a report. It is also helpful to know that reports will probably include the following abbreviations: OD (abbreviation for *oculus dexter*, or right eye), OS (abbreviation for *oculus sinister*, or left eye), and OU (abbreviation for *oculus uterque*, or both eyes). Parents and professionals should not hesitate to request a detailed explanation of any evaluation report that is not clearly understood.

Assessment of cognitive visual perceptual disorders

Visual perception is a broad term used to describe a wide array of cognitive processes involved in understanding visual information once it reaches the brain, relating it to other sensory information and past experiences, and using that information to solve problems and make decisions. The more common types of visual perception problems have been described in the previous chapter.

Children with autism, AD/HD, and other learning disabilities, have a high incidence of visual perception problems. They often have difficulty recognizing, remembering, organizing and interpreting visual images. As a result, they are easily confused in situations that involve using written or pictorial symbols for learning. The relationship of visual perception problems to reading disorders is well understood, but children with these problems also have difficulty with other symbolic learning, such as the use of graphs, charts, tables, measurements, etc. They may also have a poor sense of direction and get lost easily, or have difficulty coordinating body movements in time and space, resulting in clumsiness. They may have difficulty recognizing non-verbal aspects of social interaction, and as a result may have difficulty negotiating friendships and communication with others.

Visual perception problems and visual efficiency problems are closely interrelated, and may be difficult to distinguish from one another. Problems with eye teaming or other aspects of binocular vision may send confusing messages to the brain, causing distorted perception. Or, distorted perception at the level of the brain may cause the child to use inefficient eye control because his or her brain has interpreted the need to look at things differently. Thus, both visual efficiency skills and visual perception skills must be looked at when considering treatment options for children who struggle to learn.

Professionals representing a wide range of training and background experiences may offer testing of visual perception skills. The professionals most often involved in this type of testing include psychologists, occupational therapists, and special educators. It is important to recognize that professionals who are in a position to test children may have varying levels of training and expertise. For example, all optometrists have some training in visual skills training and may offer these services as part of their practice, but those who have completed post-doctoral training and certification are more likely to have expertise in this area. Table 4.2 presents an overview of the training and typical approaches of various professionals who may be responsible for testing a child's visual perception skills.

Some evaluators will provide a more in-depth assessment than others, and some will use results to foster recommendations about potential intervention approaches, while others will test more for diagnostic purposes only. Of the professionals described in Table 4.2, *occupational therapists* are the most likely to offer direct instructional intervention for visual perception problems that have been identified through testing, while *special educators* and *reading specialists* will commonly incorporate strategies to compensate for perceptual problems into more traditional educational interventions.

Occupational therapists are health care professionals who address problems with fine motor and perceptual development that interfere with self-care, play, and learning, which are the primary occupations of children. Occupational therapists have a Master's degree that includes broad training that is often more medically based than that of other professionals who typically evaluate visual perception. They have skills for recognizing the symptoms of and screening for functional vision difficulties, and may work in collaboration with developmental/behavioral optometrists to provide a coordinated program of intervention. Many occupational therapists who choose to specialize in pediatric practice also have advanced training in a method called *sensory integration therapy*, which is an approach that helps children to improve the way

Table 4.2 Professionals involved in assessment of visual perception problems

Professional	Focus of assessment	Qualifications	Indications
Behavioral optometrist	• Problems with eye health, refraction, or visual efficiency impacting perception	• Doctor of Optometry • Advanced training in children's vision skills • Board certification (desirable) available through American Academy of Optometry (Diplomates), or Fellow of College of Optometrists in Vision Development (FCOVD)	• Physical or behavioral signs and symptoms of vision difficulties
Developmental pediatrician	• Medical diagnosis of developmental, learning, and behavioral disorders	• Medical degree • Board certification in pediatrics • Three-year post-doctoral fellowship in developmental pediatrics	• Unknown etiology or complications of developmental disabilities • Conflict of opinions regarding diagnosis or treatment
Neuro-psychologist	• In-depth evaluation of the brain's ability to perform a variety of cognitive and functional tasks	• Doctoral degree in psychology • Licensure (varies by state) • Supervised post-doctoral training in neuropsychology • Board certification in neuropsychology through American Board of Professional Psychology (desirable)	• Comprehensive evaluation of mental function, including intelligence, attention, memory, perception, and learning ability • Often conducted to determine the impact of illness or disability on brain function
Neurologist	• Medical diagnosis of nervous system disorders	• Medical degree • Residency in pediatric neurology • Board certification in pediatric neurology (desirable)	• Loss or plateau of skill • Unknown etiology of problems • Medication for AD/HD or other behaviors
Occupational therapist	• Sensory-motor aspects of learning, including visual perception, as they impact daily living skills	*Occupational therapist* • B.S. or M.S. degree in occupational therapy • Board certification (NBCOT) • Licensure (varies by state)	• Poor vision skills • Non-verbal learning delays • Poor motor skills • Limited success with daily living activities

Table 4.2 cont.

Professional	Focus of assessment	Qualifications	Indications
Occupational therapist *cont.*		• Advanced training/ certification in pediatrics or sensory integration (desirable) *Occupational Therapy Assistant (OTA)* • AS in occupational therapy • Board certification (NBCOT) • Licensure (varies by state) • Must have direct supervision from an occupational therapist	• Task avoidance, poor attention, problems with social interactions
Pediatrician	• Medical problems affecting learning and behavior; screening of developmental milestones	• Board certified pediatrician	• Primary care provider • Refers to other specialists as appropriate • Medication
Psychologist	• Overall intelligence • Visual perception relative to other cognitive skills • Emotional/behavioral concerns	*Psychologist* • Doctoral degree • Internship and fellowship (varies by state) • State licensure *School psychologist* • Master's degree • Supervised field training • State licensure • National certification (NCSP)	
Special educator or Reading specialist	• Academic achievement and contributing factors • Learning style	• Minimum Bachelor's degree in education • Supervised student teaching • Special certifications (e.g., Early childhood, Special education, Reading specialist) vary by state	• Academic underachievement

that they interpret sensory information, including vision, for more effective learning and behavioral regulation.

Over the years, many tests have been developed to assess the visual perception abilities of children. Table 4.3 describes some of the more commonly used tests for children with autism, AD/HD, or learning disabilities. Some of these are designed to evaluate visual perception skills alone, while others include subtests that relate to visual perception as part of a more comprehensive battery. It is important to be aware that tests are often revised over time, and may exist in multiple versions. This is done either to modify the procedures in accordance with new scientific information, or to update the normative data consistent with changes in the comparative population. Where revisions have occurred, Table 4.3 lists only the most current version of each test. All of the tests described in Table 4.3 can be purchased through one of the test publishers listed in the resource section at the end of this book.

Table 4.3 Tests commonly used to evaluate visual perception in children

Name of test	Description
Bender Visual-Motor Gestalt Test, Second Edition (2003). Riverside Publishing	• Ages three through adult • Testing time five to ten minutes, plus five minutes for supplemental tests • Brief assessment of visual-motor integration that includes simple supplemental tests of motor and perceptual ability, as well as visual-motor memory
Benton Visual Retention Test, Fifth Edition (1992). The Psychological Corporation	• Children through adults • Testing time five minutes • Assesses visual perception, visual memory, and visuoconstructive abilities
Beery VMI, Fifth Edition (2004). Modern Curriculum Press	• Ages two through 18 years 11 months • Testing time 10–15 minutes, plus five minutes for each supplemental subtest • Assesses visual-motor skills through a form copy task. Supplemental visual perception and motor subtests are available
Comprehensive Test of Visual Functioning (1995). Slosson Educational Publications, Inc	• Ages eight and older • Testing time 25 minutes • Detects visual processing problems using the following scales: visual acuity, visual tracking, figure–ground, visual closure, spatial orientation, perceptual reasoning, visual-motor, reading decoding, and thematic maturity

Table 4.3 cont.

Name of test	Description
Developmental Test of Visual Perception, Second Edition (1993). Pro-Ed, Inc	• Ages four through ten; adolescent/adult version available for ages 11–74 • Testing time 30 to 60 minutes • Eight subtests measure eye hand coordination, copying, spatial relations, position in space, figure–ground, visual closure, visual-motor speed, and visual closure
Jordan Left/Right Reversal Test, Revised (1990). Academic Therapy Publications	• Ages five through 12 • Testing time 20 minutes, appropriate for group administration • Assesses reversals of letters, numbers, and words
Kaufman Assessment Battery for Children (K-ABC), Second Edition (2004). American Guidance Services, Inc	• Ages three through eight • Testing time 25–70 minutes • Comprehensive cognitive assessment tool that includes several subtests involving visual perceptual reasoning • Must be administered by a psychologist
Kent Visual Perceptual Test (1996). Psychological Assessment Resources, Inc	• Ages five through adult • Testing time 25–30 minutes • Assesses three visual processes related to the development of basic reading, math, and written expression: discrimination, copying, and immediate memory
Motor-Free Visual Perception Test (MVPT-III), Third edition (2002). Academic Therapy Publications	• Ages four through 85 • Testing time 20 minutes • Measures visual perception without demanding a motor response. Tasks include matching, figure–ground, closure, visual memory, and form discrimination
Neitz Test of Color Vision (2001). Western Psychological Services	• Ages pre-kindergarten through adult • Testing time less than five minutes • Quick, reliable method for screening for color blindness, can be group-administered
NEPSY®: A Developmental Neuropsychological Assessment (1997). The Psychological Corporation	• Ages three through 12 • Testing time variable • Series of neuropsychological subtests that assess attention and executive functions, language and communication, sensorimotor functions, visual-spatial functions, and learning and memory • Must be administered by a psychologist
Preschool Visual Motor Integration Assessment (2001). Therapro Inc	• Ages three-and-a-half through five-and-a-half • Testing time 20 minutes • Consists of two subtests, drawing and block patterns, that address a variety of perceptual skills including perception of position in space, awareness of spatial relationships, color and shape discrimination, matching two attributes simultaneously, and the ability to reproduce what is seen

Continued on next page

Table 4.3 cont.

Name of test	Description
Sensory Integration and Praxis Tests (SIPT) Ayres (1989). Western Psychological Services	• Ages four through eight years 11 months • Testing time two hours • Measures the sensory integration processes that underlie learning. Seventeen subtests measure visual, tactile, and kinesthetic perception as well as motor performance • Must be certified to administer this test (usually occupational therapist)
Stanford-Binet Intelligence Scales, Fifth Edition (2003). Riverside Publishing	• Ages two through adult • Testing time variable • Comprehensive measure of intelligence that includes assessment of visual-spatial processing, and allows the comparison of verbal to non-verbal cognitive reasoning • Must be administered by a psychologist
Test of Visual-Perceptual Skills (non-motor)—Revised (TVPS-R) (1996). Academic Therapy Publications	• Ages four through 13; upper level version (TVPS-UL) available for ages 12 through 18 • Testing time 10–20 minutes • Comprehensive test of visual perceptual skills without relying on a motor response. Provides an overall score as well as subtest scores in the following areas: visual discrimination, visual memory, visual-spatial relationships, visual form constancy, visual sequential memory, visual figure–ground, and visual closure
Wechsler Preschool and Primary Scale of Intelligence, Third Edition (WPPSI-III) (2002).	• Ages two years six months through seven years three months • Testing time 30–60 minutes • Comprehensive measure of intelligence in young children • Must be administered by a psychologist
Wechsler Intelligence Scale for Children, Fourth Edition (WISC-IV) (2003).	• Ages six through 16 • Testing time 65–80 minutes • Provides a measure of intellectual functioning for general and specific cognitive abilities, including perceptual reasoning • Must be administered by a psychologist
Wide Range Assessment of Memory and Learning, Second Edition (2003). Psychological Assessment Resources, Inc	• Ages five through adult • Testing time 60 minutes for core battery, with additional subtests available to supplement the core battery • Evaluates both immediate and delayed memory, including two visual memory subtests

When choosing which test or tests to use, professionals attempt to identify well-designed tools that will help them to make the best possible clinical decisions. Because no test is perfect, scores should not be used to make clinical decisions unless they are consistent with clinical observations of the child's functional performance and with the clinician's overall impression of the child. Tests may be described as either criterion-referenced, or standardized. Criterion-referenced tests measure the child's performance according to an established standard, and are used more for descriptive purposes than as a true measure of ability. Standardized tests are tests that have been developed so that procedures, materials, and scoring techniques are used in exactly the same way each time the test is given. This ensures that there is uniformity across test subjects. In a standardized test, the child's score can be compared with those obtained by a group of test subjects who have comparable qualities (age, grade level, socioeconomic status, etc.). By looking at the scores obtained on standardized tests, the examiner can see how the child is performing relative to other children his or her age. To meaningfully interpret test scores, they must also be analyzed in relation to other measures of the child's cognitive abilities, especially measures of overall intelligence or language functioning. This is done to determine whether low scores on visual perception tasks are indicative of generally limited intelligence, or represent a more specific perceptual disorder. Table 4.4 provides a description of different types of test scores that may be included in an evaluation report.

There are a number of ways for parents to obtain testing of visual perception skills in children who are suspected of having these problems. In the United States, federal legislation (Education of the Handicapped Act Amendments of 1986, or Public Law 99–457, Part H) provides for free early intervention services for children up to age three who meet eligibility requirements, which vary from state to state. Screening for visual perception problems is usually conducted when children are considered for eligibility, and more comprehensive evaluation of visual perception skills may occur if problems are suspected. These tests are usually conducted by an occupational therapist, or in some cases a psychologist. Children who are identified as having visual perception disorders may or may not be eligible for early intervention services, such as free occupational therapy, through this system.

Federal legislation (the Individuals with Disabilities Education Act (IDEA), or Public Law 101–476 of 1990 and its amendments made in 1997 and 2004) also provides for free special education and support services to children ages 3–21 with special needs. In most states, the local school district is responsible for providing these services. Children with disabilities including visual perception disorders may be eligible for services, including occupational therapy, if they meet the local school district's eligibility requirements for classification as a special education student. However, parents must recognize that these services may be limited in their scope.

Table 4.4 Understanding test scores

Score	Description
Raw Score	The number of test items the subject completed successfully. In a criterion-referenced test, the raw score may be reported or reported as the percentage of items passed. For standardized tests, the raw score has little meaning until it has been converted using a variety of statistical procedures.
Percentile	The percentage of scores that were below the child's score. If the child scored at the 75th percentile, he or she scored as well or better than 75% of children in the normative group. A drawback in using percentiles is that there is inequality between percentile units, with a larger difference at the ends of the scale than in the middle. Therefore, there is a greater difference in performance between the 90th and 95th percentile than there is between the 50th and 55th percentile.
Standard Deviation (S.D.)	A numerical index that indicates how widely spread the scores were for the normative group. In a normally distributed bell curve, 68.3% of subjects will score within one standard deviation of the mean (-1.0 S.D. to +1.0 S.D.), and 95.4% will score within two standard deviations of the mean (-2.0 to +2.0).
Standard Scores	There are a number of different formulas for using the standard deviation to convert to different types of standard scores. For example, a standard score may be based upon a mean of 100 and a standard deviation of 15, meaning that scores ranging from 85–100 are considered average. A *T-Score* is a type of standard score adjusted to have a mean of 50 and a standard deviation of 10, so scores ranging from 40–60 would be considered average. A *stanine* is a standard score with a range of 1–9, where 5 is the mean and the standard deviation is 2. Thus, stanines of 3–7 are considered average.
Age Equivalent Scores	The average age of children in the normative group who achieved the same raw score as the child. Although age equivalent scores seem easy to understand, they are easily over-interpreted. A major limitation is that most skills measured by tests do not increase incrementally by the same amount each year. For example, most children show more gains in gross motor skills between the ages of one and two than between the ages of 15 and 16.

Source: Reprinted with permission from Kurtz, L.A. (2003) *How to Help a Clumsy Child: Strategies for Young Children with Developmental Motor Concerns.* London: Jessica Kingsley Publishers, p.46.

Only those therapy services needed to support the student's educational needs are provided for under this legislation. Typically, frequency and intensity of therapy, as well as the amount of direct parent instruction, are more limited than may be available through hospitals or other providers of therapy such as private clinics. For this reason, some parents choose to supplement programs offered through the school with private outpatient therapy. Parents and teachers should also be aware that there is additional federal legislation that may enable a school-aged student with a disability to receive evaluation and treatment of visual perception disorders through the local school district even if they are not eligible to receive special education services. Upon parent request, students with an identified disability may be eligible for services and accommodations, including occupational therapy, under entitlements defined by the Americans with Disabilities Act (ADA) of 1990, Section 504 of the Rehabilitation Act of 1973, or state regulations governing the education of students. Parents may request this testing if they believe that their child's disability limits his or her participation in daily activities at school.

Finally, testing by an occupational therapist or other professional may be covered by medical insurance in settings outside of the school. One advantage to using private resources for evaluation is that it may provide a more comprehensive and detailed evaluation than that which can be provided by public schools.

When any form of intervention is undertaken, parents are encouraged to be active participants in the program. This is more difficult to achieve when the intervention takes place at school as opposed to a private outpatient setting, but is important nonetheless. Parents should contribute to setting goals that are meaningful to them, and should have a clear understanding of the methods and timelines anticipated for achieving those goals.

Regardless of the intervention that is recommended for the child, whether it be vision therapy, special education, occupational therapy, or other services, it is important for parents to be vigilant about continually evaluating whether the intervention is effectively meeting their child's needs. Unfortunately, the quality and commitment of schools, clinics, and professionals can vary greatly. Also, a child's individual needs will change over time as he or she grows and matures. The list below offers some guidelines for evaluating the quality of any intervention program for children with special learning needs:

Desirable qualities in an intervention program

The professional:

- treats you and your child with respect
- sets a positive tone during sessions
- has the appropriate training and experience
- communicates regularly and in a way you can understand
- includes you in all decisions regarding your child
- willingly communicates with other professionals involved with your child
- knows what (s)he can/cannot accomplish, helping you find other help if necessary
- is effective in helping your child to learn.

The program:

- is based on principles that have been explained to you
- includes specific goals that you understand and have agreed upon
- includes a projected time frame for achievement of goals
- provides regular, written reports of progress and current recommendations
- includes home/school recommendations that are realistic to manage.

The environment:

- is clean and safe
- includes a wide variety of appropriate materials for intervention.

The child:

- relates well with the professional, and finds most activities enjoyable
- makes observable changes in performance or behavior.

Source: Adapted with permission from Kurtz, L.A. (2003) *How to Help a Clumsy Child: Strategies for Young Children with Developmental Motor Concerns.* London: Jessica Kingsley Publishers, p.48.

References

Americans with Disabilities Act (ADA) of 1990, P.L. 101–336, 42 U.S.C. §§ 12101 *et seq.*

Education of the Handicapped Act Amendments of 1986, P.L. 99–457, 20 U.S.C. §§ 1400 *et seq.*

Individuals with Disabilities Education Act (IDEA) of 1990, P.L. 101–476, 20 U.S.C. §§ 1400 *et seq.*

Individuals with Disabilities Education Act (IDEA) Amendments of 1997, P.L. 105–17, 20 U.S.C. §§ 1400 *et seq.*

Individuals with Disabilities Education Improvement Act (IDEIA) of 2004, P.L. 108–446, 20 U.S.C. §§ 1400 *et seq.*

Rehabilitation Act of 1973, P.L. 93–112, 29 U.S.C. §§ 701 *et seq.*

Chapter 5

ACTIVITIES FOR IMPROVING VISUAL SKILLS

The following sections describe suggested activities that may be used at home, in school, or in therapeutic settings to support the development of visual skills. They are in no way intended to replace the need for professional evaluation by a developmental/behavioral optometrist and/or an occupational therapist or other specialist when vision difficulties are suspected. They are also not intended for use as a substitute for vision therapy that occurs under the supervision of a professional. However, with guidance from the appropriate professionals, these activities may be of interest to parents, teachers, and others who work with children who have either functional vision problems, or visual perception problems that impact learning and daily living skills. Effort has been made to select activities that do not require the purchase of expensive materials and equipment. Suggestions for constructing some simple equipment has been provided in the appendix included at the end of this book.

When introducing a program of vision development activities to a child, there are several important considerations to keep in mind:

- The children must have some understanding of the purpose of participating in special activities, so that he or she will feel motivated to put good effort into the activities. It is often helpful to think about what kinds of daily occurrences are frustrating to the child, and to build your explanation around these frustrations. For younger children, very simple statements will suffice, for example, "These games will help your eyes to get stronger so that you can learn to read more easily." Older children appreciate being given truthful yet simplified descriptions of the type of vision difficulty they have, and why it makes certain activities difficult or tiring.

- The amount of time spent in working on vision activities is less important than the quality of the time spent. If you can, try to set aside 10 to 15 minutes two to three times per week to focus on structured activities, varying the activities as needed to maintain the child's attention and effort. Often, it is also possible to embed activities that support vision development into the child's daily routine, once you have an understanding of the skills that need to be strengthened. For example, sorting through the laundry to find matching pairs of socks is an excellent activity for strengthening visual figure–ground and discrimination skills, and cleaning windows can be an excellent way to promote visual scanning to look for spots and streaks. Looking for birds on a nature walk, license plates during a long road trip, or shells on the beach, are other simple ways of strengthening visual skills.

- Activities should always take place in an atmosphere that is positive and playful. This will help the child to stay engaged with the activity, and to work at his or her best. Offer praise for good effort, or if necessary, reward effort with stars or stickers to be traded for a tangible reward. Often, the child's reaction to a particular activity can serve as a measure of the appropriateness of the activity. If the child becomes easily bored, the activity probably does not pose enough challenge to be helpful, and should be graded up to a higher level of difficulty. If the child becomes very frustrated, the activity is probably too hard, and should be dropped until the child's skill level increases.

- Consult with the professionals involved in the care of the child to determine whether activities are best done with one or both eyes, and with glasses on or off.

Activities to improve functional vision

The following activities are designed to help children develop skills related to ocular motility, binocular coordination, and eye hand coordination. Because these are all skills that relate to muscular coordination of the eyes during functional activities, it is helpful to have some understanding of the basic principles by which children develop muscular coordination skills.

One of the most important factors in how children develop motor control is the way in which they use their various senses to guide their learning. Most people are familiar with the senses of sight, hearing, touch, smell and taste, and have at least a general appreciation for how these senses might help children to learn. Obviously, children need to see and recognize the shapes of letters if they are to read, and must hear and understand words if they are to communicate. However, there are other important senses that are felt on a more subconscious level, and are therefore not as well understood.

The *vestibular* sense is designed to provide the brain with information about gravity and motion, and plays a role in developing balance as well as helping to coordinate movements of the eyes, head and body. Located within the inner ear, it contains two types of receptors. The *otoliths* consist of tiny crystals attached to hair-like nerves that move in response to gravity, vibration, or subtle changes in head position, thus sending impulses to the brain. Also, each ear contains three sets of *semicircular canals* that are filled with fluid as well as hair-like cells, each oriented in a different direction. Rapid motion, such as that produced by jumping, rolling down a hill, or riding down a hill on a sled, causes the fluid to surge through one or more of the canals, disrupting the position of the hair-nerves and sending information about the nature of the motion to the brain. Sensation from the vestibular system influences many other aspects of a child's behavior and learning, therefore contributing to development in many ways. For example, it helps to promote an alert state needed for learning, contributes to the coordination of eye movements, helps the two sides of the body coordinate their movements, and influences muscle tone throughout the body.

The *proprioceptive* system is perhaps equally important to the development of motor skills. It is a complex anatomical system consisting of various receptors located in the joints, muscles, and tendons that provide the child with a subconscious awareness of body position and body movements. For example, if you were to suddenly close your eyes, you could still "feel" whether your arms are crossed in front of your chest, hanging down by your side, or resting in your lap. Proprioceptive sensations are constantly bombarding the brain, providing the information needed to allow subtle adjustments to body positions as we move. For example, imagine that you are getting ready for your morning shower, and step into the tub leading with your right foot. It is your vision that tells the brain whether your right foot is aimed in the right direction, and whether it will land inside the shower stall. However, to maintain balance during the movement, your body also needs to shift weight to the left leg and tilt the trunk slightly to the left. Without any conscious effort on your part, proprioceptive input from the leg and trunk combined with a visual image tell the brain how much adjustment is not too much or too little, but just right.

Because of the relationship of these senses to developing eye muscle coordination, it is important to involve them when designing vision exercises. In general, exercises that focus on improving functional vision skills are most challenging when they are physically active, involving large muscle coordination and total body awareness. The difficulty level of eye exercises, therefore, can be increased by challenging the child's balance and postural stability during these activities. For this reason, once the child can perform an activity successfully while in a sitting or standing position, the challenge can be increased by performing the activity while standing on an uneven surface (such as sand or grass), sitting on a large ball or one-legged balance stool, or by using a balance beam or balance board. These items are available commercially and are usually present in clinical settings, but can be made inexpensively at home as well. A simple two-inch by four-inch plank that has been sanded to avoid splinters can serve as a balance beam. Instructions for making a balance board and a one-legged balance stool are included in the appendix. The following activities are suggested to promote the development of functional vision skills:

- *Target games.* Throwing balls, rings, darts, etc. at targets at various distances from the eyes. Increase the difficulty by increasing the distance between targets, increasing the speed of throwing, or by challenging balance.

- *Paddle balls.* Bouncing a ball up in the air using a paddle can greatly help eye hand coordination. This can be done by the child alone, counting the number of "hits" before the ball is dropped, or with a partner. Start with using a paddle to hit a slow-moving balloon, and increase the difficulty to hitting a faster-moving ball such as a koosh ball or ping-pong ball. The child can use just one paddle, or can hold a paddle in each hand, hitting the ball back and forth between the two hands. A simple paddle for use with a balloon can be made by bending a wire clothes hanger into a paddle shape, pulling the leg of a pair of panty hose over the wide part of the paddle, and holding the panty hose in place by wrapping the handle with several lengths of duct tape. See Figure 5.1.

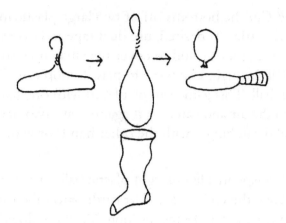

Figure 5.1: Clothes hanger paddle

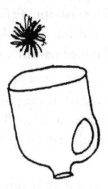

Figure 5.2: Bottle scoop

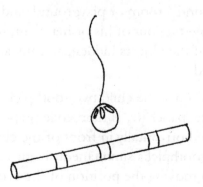

Figure 5.3: Stick and ball game

- *Scoop ball.* Cut the bottoms off of two large plastic milk bottles or detergent bottles. If desired, use duct tape to cover the cut edges so that they are smooth, and to cover the small hole so that objects cannot fall through. Use these to play "scoop catch" with a beanbag or koosh ball. This game can be played with one hand (tossing the ball up in the air and catching it again), with two hands (tossing the ball up and catching it with the other hand) or with a partner. See Figure 5.2.

- *Stick ball.* Suspend a lightweight plastic ball on a string from the ceiling. Give the child a dowel or cardboard tube from wrapping paper approximately 18 inches long. Mark the dowel with colored bands, using a marker or colored tape (e.g., red on the right end, blue on the left end, and yellow in the middle). Ask the child to tap the ball smoothly and rhythmically using the middle (yellow) part of the dowel. Gradually increase the difficulty by having the child tap out "patterns" such as red-blue-red-blue, etc. This requires considerable eye hand coordination and bilateral coordination. See Figure 5.3.

- *Flashlight tag.* Sitting in a dark room, move a flashlight in a random pattern while the child uses another flashlight to keep up with your path. Gradually increase the speed of the game, and the size of the area used.

- *Flashlight match.* Sitting in a dark room, use a flashlight to "draw" shapes, letters, or words onto a distant wall, while the child guesses what has been drawn.

- *Hide and seek for the eyes.* Hide small objects, such as marbles or dominoes, around a room or playground, and ask the child to find them without getting out of his or her chair, using only the eyes. Vary the size of the objects hidden, and the amount of contrast to the background.

- *Toothpick tunnel.* Give the child two toothpicks, one for each hand. Hold a cylinder (paper towel tube, toilet paper tube, or plastic drinking straw) horizontally in front of the child, and ask him or her to place both toothpicks simultaneously into each end of the cylinder. Keep moving the position of the cylinder as the child places the toothpicks in and out of the straw. See Figure 5.4.

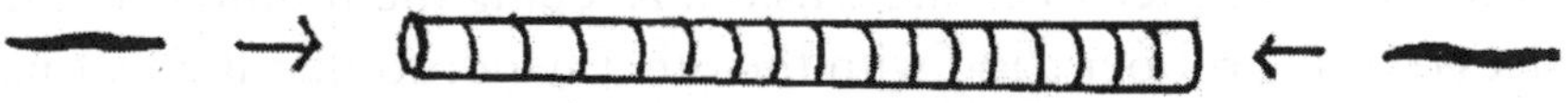

Figure 5.4: Toothpick tunnel

- *Fishing.* Using a dowel or wrapping paper tube, tie a 24-inch string to one end with a small magnet at the end of the string. Draw letters or shapes on both sides of three-inch by five-inch index cards, and place a paper clip on each card. Have the child "fish" for the cards, especially when in a balance-challenged position.

- *Puff ball.* Using a straw and a ping-pong ball, cotton ball, or small piece of tissue paper, have the child blow through the straw to move the ball through a maze or obstacle course.

- *Domino race track.* Teach the child to line up dominoes into complex patterns, then knock down the first domino and visually track the progress of the dominoes falling down.

- *Private eyes.* Take a page from a magazine or book (number of lines and size of print depending on the child's age). Teach the child to be a "detective" by tracing each line from left to right with a pencil, and looking for specified items. For example, have the child cross out all the "t's," or circle each word beginning with "b," without skipping any lines or letters.

- *Mazes, dot-to-dot, and labyrinth games.* These are all types of activities that help to develop eye hand coordination skills. The larger the size, the more work for the eyes to follow along.

- *Button box.* Cut off the bottom of an egg carton, and mark each compartment with different colors, shapes, or letters. Have the child attempt to toss a button from one compartment to another.

- *Flying bands.* Teach the child how to "shoot" a rubber band at targets that have been placed at various distances. Start by extending the thumb, loop the rubber band around the tip of the thumb, and pull it towards the face to create tension. Keeping the thumb extended, let go of the rubber band with the other hand, so that it flies forward towards the target.

- *Marble catch.* Using an empty coffee can with a plastic lid, cut a hole in the center of the lid, just large enough for a marble. Have the child sit on a large ball or one-legged stool, and "catch" marbles as they are rolled towards him or her. The child picks up each marble and places it in the hole of the can. Increase the difficulty level by rolling more than one marble at a time, so that the child has to shift eye position to keep track of the multiple targets. See Figure 5.5.

- *Marble mazes.* Create simple mazes onto a flat surface, such as a rectangular piece of cardboard, or a styrofoam tray used by supermarkets to package meats. Using a hot glue gun, trace the lines of a maze so that they are slightly raised. Have the child hold the tray with both hands, and try to guide a marble through the maze.

- *Hole in one.* Attach a length of string to a ping-pong ball (poke a small hole in the ball and use hot glue to adhere the string). Tie the other end of the string to one end of a paper towel tube, and teach the child to try to "catch" the ball with the tube. Increasing the length of the string enhances the challenge. See Figure 5.6.

- *Zoom ball.* These can be purchased commercially, or can be inexpensively homemade as follows. Cut two nine- to 10-foot lengths of a slippery cord. Next, tie each end of each cord so that there are now two cords, each with a handle on both ends. Thread two handles through a toilet tissue tube. Two people stand facing each other holding onto the handles, at a distance that causes the cords to be taut. As one person brings his or her arms together, the other brings his or her hands apart. If the cords are kept taut and the timing is correct, the paper tube will "zoom" back and forth, creating a good opportunity to practice convergent eye movements. See Figure 5.7.

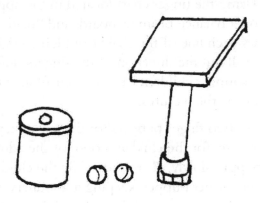

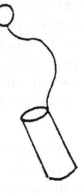

Figure 5.5: Marble can and balance stool

Figure 5.6: Hole in one game

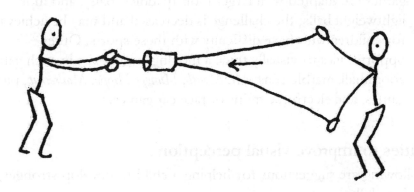

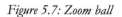

Figure 5.7: Zoom ball

- *Finger chart.* Using the finger chart located in the appendix, have the child stand on a balance beam or board, and "read" the fingers as he or she follows each line of the chart from left to right. Older children can call out the direction of the fingers (left, right, up, down) while younger children can use their fingers to point in the same direction as the pictures.

- *Finger pals.* Use two finger puppets (or draw a smiley face on the tip of the finger), one for the child and one for the adult. The adult moves the puppet slowly all around, while the child attempts to follow with his or her puppet, keeping it about six inches from the adult's puppet. Every now and then, the adult says "Give me a kiss (or hug, or high five)", and the child touches his or her puppet to the adult's puppet.

- *Spoon relay.* Provide the child with a plastic spoon and a cotton ball or ping-pong ball. Ask the child to balance the ball on the spoon while holding the handle of the spoon in his or her mouth, then balancing it while walking on a balance beam or through a simple obstacle course. This requires the child to frequently shift visual focus from the spoon (near vision) to the feet (distant vision) in order to balance.

- *Commercial sports and games.* Many games and activities are commercially available that can help children to develop better eye hand coordination. Sports that involve using a ball or other projectile (golf, bowling, badminton, T-ball, tetherball, ping-pong, frisbee) all help to develop vision skills. In general, when these games are adapted with larger tools (paddles, bats), and more lightweight balls, the challenge is decreased and may be achievable for children who have difficulty with these sports. Other opportunities to visually track a moving target exist in such games as zoom ball, marble runs, *Mr. Mouth*, *Hungry Hippo*, *Mousetrap*, pinball games, and electronic trains or race car games.

Activities to improve visual perception

The following are suggestions for helping a child to develop stronger visual perception skills:

Visual discrimination

- Practice sorting shapes by shape, color, size, or other attribute.

- Practice nesting cups or dolls to develop size discrimination.

- String beads according to color or shape sequence on a picture.

- Have the child identify objects in a room that are of a certain shape, for example, circles = clock, face, ball, wheels; rectangle = window, tabletop, light switch cover.

- Bingo or lotto games using colors or shapes.

- Puzzles.

- Practice making shapes, letters, or designs using toothpicks, drinking straws, popsicle sticks, or cotton swabs.

- Find a large, intricately detailed picture in a magazine, and have the child find all the "tall" things, "small" things, "round" things, "blue" things, etc.

- Cut out individual pictures of objects from magazines, then trace these onto construction paper so that you have a silhouette of the picture. Have the child match the silhouette to the picture.

- Trace a letter or shape on the child's back, using your finger. Have the child guess the shape, then lie on the floor and try to make the shape using his or her body.

Visual figure-ground discrimination

- Purchase "hidden picture" books and games, for example, *Where's Waldo?*

- Go on a treasure hunt in a cluttered room and find a list of small objects that have been hidden.

- Jigsaw puzzles.

- Cut a section of print from a newspaper or magazine. Have the child go on a "treasure hunt" and circle all the words that begin or end with a targeted letter or letter combination (e.g., all the words that start with "th" or end with "s").

- Trace shapes or letters on a piece of paper so that they overlap. Then have the child trace each shape using a different colored crayon.

- Make pictures of shapes or letters with missing parts for the child to complete.

Perception of spatial relationships

- Copy block design patterns (e.g., mosaic, parquetry, tanagrams, etc.).

- Copy pegboard designs from a pattern (e.g., *Lite-Brite*).

- Dot-to-dot pictures and mazes.

- Provide various crafts or models that require the child to copy directions from a visual model.

- Create an obstacle course and draw a simple map to illustrate the course. Place the drawing inside of a plastic sheet protector, then use a wipe-off marker to draw a path for the child to follow.

- Read a comic strip to the child, then cut apart the segments and have the child re-arrange the story in the correct order.

- Teach the child to set the table, remembering the correct location of utensils, napkins, cups, etc.

- Teach the child to remember directions for getting to familiar places, such as the playground, and to use the words "right" and "left" when describing how to get to these places.

- Take a cardboard paper tube, and place two or more blocks of different colors inside the tube, one at a time. Play a game of tipping the tube to the right or left, or rotating it completely before tipping. Have the child predict the order of blocks to come out of the tube when tipped.

- Tie a red ribbon around the child's right wrist, and a blue ribbon around the left wrist. Teach the child that red is for the right hand, because they both start with "R." Tie ribbons around your own wrists, but on opposite sides so that if you sit facing the child, red will match red and blue will match blue. Teach the child to imitate different rhythmic patterns, such as "red, red, blue," or "red, both,

both, blue." As skill increases, take off the ribbons and teach the child to follow patterns using only the words "right, left, and both."

- Draw a green line down the left-hand margin of the page, and a red line down the right-hand margin, to remind the child where to begin and end writing.

- Teach the child to leave a finger space between words when writing. Consider offering a "finger buddy" made by drawing a smiley face on one end of a craft stick to use in place of a finger.

- Use graph paper to help the child line up number columns when doing math computation.

Visual memory

- Show the child a group of objects, then cover with a cloth and remove one object. The child must identify which object was removed.

- Show the child a group of objects, then cover with a cloth and add one object. The child must identify the new object.

- Create a design with blocks, beads, pegs, or crayons. Hide the design, and ask the child to copy it from memory.

- Line up a series of objects, and ask the child to identify the order from left to right. Have the child hide his or her eyes while you change the order of the objects. The child must reproduce the correct order.

- Use playing cards or commercial memory game cards that are placed face down on the table. The child and a partner take turns turning over two cards to find a "match." Start by placing cards in straight rows. The difficulty level is increased when cards are placed randomly on the table.

- Show the child a detailed picture from a magazine or book for about ten seconds. Then have the child list all of the items he or she can remember.

Spatial organizational skills

- Teach the child to prepare for school the night before. Create a checklist that helps plan what he or she will wear, check to see that homework is completed, and pack the backpack with necessary items.

- Provide a daily schedule for the child to review and refer to throughout the day. Designate a person (adult or peer) to help the child review his or her schedule at designated checkpoints throughout the day.

- Teach the child to organize his or her desk so that materials are placed in the same location each time they are put away. If necessary, prepare a simple diagram to provide visual reference. Use color-coded folders to help sort papers into various subject areas.

- Establish daily routines, such as cleaning out the backpack, with clear, concise rules (e.g., first, things to take home and give to parents; second, things to put away or throw away; third, things that require action and must be returned to school).

- In the classroom, post charts that visually outline expected classroom rules and procedures (e.g., at start of day, before you go home, etc.).

- Provide checklists for the student to self-check assignment completion.

- Provide advance warning when routines must be disrupted or changed.

- Assist the child to develop plans of how he or she will complete long-term assignments, with a schedule for completion of small steps needed to reach the goal.

- Leave time at the end of the day for organizing materials and checking to see if homework assignments are clearly understood.

- Allow calculators and digital watches for children who need them.

Chapter 6

HELPING CHILDREN TO COMPENSATE FOR PROBLEMS WITH VISION

When a child has difficulty with functional vision or perceptual skills, it is important to recognize the impact of these difficulties on all aspects of daily living. A person's eyes are used during virtually all waking hours, and when the eyes do not work efficiently, eye strain and frustration are the likely result. Also, in today's culture, many children spend less time in active, outdoor play, and more time watching television, using a computer, or playing video games, all of which involve intense visual focus at a near point. This poses a greater risk for developing eyestrain. Besides providing professional evaluation and interventions such as glasses, therapy, or special education for children with vision problems, it is also important to consider accommodations to the home and school environments that may help to reduce the demands on the visual system. Suggestions are provided as two categories: 1. those that are designed to promote good visual hygiene and are therefore useful for all children, and 2. strategies that may help to compensate for specific visual problems, and that should be selected in consultation with a professional. For children enrolled in special education programs, these strategies may need to be included as specific modifications to the child's individualized educational plan (IEP).

Strategies for maintaining visual hygiene
- When doing close visual work, take frequent visual "breaks" by looking up and focusing on a distant target for about ten seconds. It

is also helpful to get up to stretch or move around at least once every 15 to 20 minutes, depending on the age of the child.

- Lighting can greatly impact the amount of stress on the visual system. Fluorescent lighting is harsher than incandescent or natural lighting. When doing close visual work, a rule of thumb is that light on the visual target should be about three times brighter than the surrounding light.

- Take care to avoid glare on work surfaces. Never place a computer or television screen directly in front of a window unless there are drapes or curtains available to block the light. Placing a blotter or large piece of dark construction paper on a desk can reduce glare from fluorescent lights.

- Try to read or do other close visual work at an eye-to-activity distance that is approximately equal to the distance between the elbow and the middle knuckles.

- Body position is important when using the eyes for close work. A chair should be of the appropriate size to promote a straight, upright posture with the feet flat on the floor. This helps both eyes to focus equally on the task at hand. Using a bookrest can help the child to maintain an upright posture when reading. Also, reading a book that is upright places less stress on the eyes than reading a book placed flat on the desk, because all of the lines of print are at an equal distance from the eyes. Discourage the child from reading, watching television, or playing video games while lying sideways on the floor, because this position causes the eyes to work asymmetrically when looking at the target.

- Television should be viewed from a distance of eight to ten feet from the screen, and while sitting upright. Take care to avoid glare on the screen from lamps or windows.

Possible compensatory strategies for vision difficulties

- Consider the best seating arrangement for the class. Sitting close to the board may help some children who have trouble maintaining focus, but may be harder for children who lack scanning skills, since they use narrower scanning movements to view the board from a distance. Seating in the middle of the classroom is optimal for many children with functional vision problems.

- Use multisensory teaching strategies and manipulatives for students who are not "natural" visual learners.

- Reduce visual distractions by providing a carrel on the desk, or placing the desk against an undecorated wall.

- For children with accommodative disorders, increase direct light onto the activity.

- For children with convergence or other binocular coordination difficulties, consider reading or performing fine motor activities while lying on the floor on the back. This allows the child to use his or her eyes while the head is supported by the floor, and may make it easier to coordinate eye movements.

- Reduce expectations for reading or copying. Either reduce the amount of work, or break it into smaller units to be done with breaks in between.

- If copying from the board is difficult, have a partner copy for the child using carbon paper, or give the child a copy of the teacher's notes to copy from.

- Teachers of young children often use widely ruled paper for penmanship in the belief that it is easier for small hands. In fact, wide-ruled paper requires more visual shift and attention, and may be harder for children with vision weaknesses. Try using paper with simple, dark or raised lines, and narrow rule.

- Reduce the amount of visual stimulation on worksheets by 1. folding the paper in half so the child looks at fewer items at a time, 2. enlarging the worksheet so that there is more white space between items, or 3. using a blank index card to hold under each item.

- Use a dark piece of construction paper under worksheets to increase the contrast.

- Use heightened visual cues to help with work organization. Examples include: 1. using a piece of masking tape to mark the correct angle for holding paper when writing, 2. yellow highlighting alternating lines to remind the child to skip every other line, 3. drawing a green line down the left margin of a page, and a red line down the right margin, to remind the child where to "start" and "stop" when writing, 4. executing math computation problems on large graph paper, to help with lining up number columns, 5. organizing work into different colored file folders so that the child can immediately find what he or she needs.

- Have the child use a finger, marker, file card with a "window" cut in the middle, or popsicle stick with a sticker on the end to prevent losing his or her place when reading.

- Reading material that is high interest and rich in pictorial cues, such as comic books, can help the child associate meaning with what is being read.

- Many computer programs are available to support the educational process. These can be highly motivating to the child, and can also often be modified for contrast, size of print, amount of stimuli on the screen, etc.

- Use word processing to limit the frustration when needing to check spelling or make other editorial changes.

- Books on tape can help the child learn to associate the written word with meaning, and can greatly increase reading fluency and comprehension in some children.

- For children who have trouble with reversals or with letter formations during writing, consider taping an alphabet guide to the desk, marking each letter with a tiny green dot to signify where the letter begins.

Chapter 7

RESOURCES

Recommended reading

(* indicates publication suitable for non-professional audiences)

*Anderson, W., Chitwood, S. and Hatden, D. (1997) *Negotiating the Special Education Maze: A Guide for Parents and Teachers, Third Edition.* Rockville, MD: Woodbine House.

*Barkley, R.A. (2000) *Taking Charge of ADHD: The Complete, Authoritative Guide for Parents, Revised Edition.* New York, NY: The Guilford Press.

*Bissell, J., Fisher, J., Owens, C. and Polcyn, P. (1988) *Sensory Motor Handbook: A Guide for Implementing and Modifying Activities in the Classroom.* Torrance, CA: Sensory Integration International.

Bundy, A.C., Lane, S. and Murray, E.A. (2002) *Sensory Integration Theory and Practice, Second Edition.* Philadelphia: F.A. Davis.

Ciuffreda, K.J. (2002) "The scientific basis for and efficacy of optometric vision therapy in nonstrabismic accommodative and vergence disorders." *Optometry 73*, 735–762.

Cooper, J. (1998) "Summary of research on the efficacy of vision therapy for specific visual dysfunctions." *The Journal of Behavioral Optometry 9*, 5, 115–119.

Efferson, L. (1995) "Disorders of vision and visual perceptual dysfunction." In D.A. Umphred (Ed.) *Neurological Rehabilitation, Third Edition.* St. Louis, MO: Mosby-Yearbook, (pp.769–801).

Gentile, M. (2005) *Functional Vision Behavior in Children: An Occupational Therapy Guide to Evaluation and Treatment Options.* Bethesda, MD: AOTA Press.

Goldstand, S., Koslowe, K.C. and Parush, S. (2005) "Vision, visual-information processing, and academic performance among seventh-grade schoolchildren: A more significant relationship than we thought?" *American Journal of Occupational Therapy 59*, 377–389.

Hellerstein, L.F. and Fishman, B. (1990) "Vision therapy and occupational therapy: An integrated approach." *Journal of Behavioral Optometry 1*, 5, 122–126.

*Hickman, L. (1992) *Songs for Sensory Integration: The Calming Tape and the Vision Tape.* Boulder, CO: Belle Curve Records.

*Hickman, L. and Hutchins, R. (2002) *Seeing Clearly: Fun Activities for Improving Visual Skills.* Las Vegas, NV: Sensory Resources.

*Kavner, R.S. (1985) *Your Child's Vision: A Parent's Guide to Seeing, Growing, and Developing.* New York, NY: Simon & Schuster, Inc.

*Kranowitz, C.S. (1998) *The Out-of-Sync Child: Recognizing and Coping with Sensory Integration Dysfunction.* New York, NY: Berkley Publishing Group.

Kurtz, L.A. (2003) *How to Help a Clumsy Child: Strategies for Young Children with Developmental Motor Concerns.* London: Jessica Kingsley Publishers.

*Lane, K.A. (1988) *Reversal Errors: Theories and Therapy Procedures.* Santa Ana, CA: Vision Extension.

*Lane, K.A. (1991) *Developing Your Child for Success.* Santa Ana, CA: Vision Extension.

*McMonnies, C.W. (1991) *A Practical Guide for Remedial Approaches to Left/Right Confusion and Reversals.* Sydney, Australia: Superior Educational Publications.

*McMonnies, C.W. (1992) *Overcoming Left/Right Confusion and Reversals: A Classroom Approach.* Sydney, Australia: Superior Educational Publications.

Miller, M.M., Menacker, S. and Batshaw, M.L. (2002) "Vision: Our window to the world." In M.L. Batshaw (Ed.) *Children with Disabilities, Fifth Edition.* Baltimore, MD: Brookes Publishing Co. (pp.165–192).

Richards, R.G. (1984) *Visual Skills Appraisal: Appraisal of Visual Performance and Coordinated Classroom Activities.* Novato, CA: Academic Therapy Publications.

Richards, R.G. (1988) *Classroom Visual Activities: A Manual to Enhance the Development of Visual Skills.* Novato, CA: Academic Therapy Publications.

Scheiman, M. (2002) *Understanding and Managing Vision Deficits: A Guide for Occupational Therapists, Second Edition.* Thorofare, NJ, Slack Inc.

Scheiman, M., Mitchell, G.L., Cotter, S., Cooper, J., Kulp, M., Rouse, M. *et al.* (2005) "The convergence insufficiency treatment trial (CITT) study group: A randomized clinical trial of treatments for convergence insufficiency in children." *Archives of Ophthalmology 123*, 14–24.

Schneck, C.M. (1998) "Lesson 5: Intervention for visual perception problems." In J. Case-Smith (Ed.) *Occupational Therapy: Making a Difference in School System Practice, A*

Self-Paced Clinical Course. Rockville, MD: American Occupational Therapy Association, Inc.

Schneck, C.M. and Lemer, P.S. (1993) "Section 5: Reading and visual perception." In C.B. Royeen (Ed.) *AOTA Self Study Series, Classroom Applications for School Based Practice*. Rockville, MD: American Occupational Therapy Association, Inc.

*Scott, E.P., Jan, J.E. and Freeman, R.D. (1985) *Can't Your Child See? A Guide for Parents of Visually Impaired Children*. Austin, TX: Pro-Ed.

*Siegel, B. (2003) *Helping Children with Autism Learn: Treatment Approaches for Parents and Professionals*. New York, NY: Oxford University Press.

*Silver, L.B. (1998) *The Misunderstood Child: Understanding and Coping with Your Child's Learning Disabilities, Third Edition*. New York, NY: Three Rivers Press.

*Trott, M.C., Laurel, M.K. and Windeck, S.L. (1993) *SenseAbilities: Understanding Sensory Integration*. Tucson, AZ: Therapy Skill Builders.

Helpful agencies, organizations, and websites

Achievers Unlimited, Inc.
104 South Main Street, Suite 417
Fond Du Lac, WI 54935-4245
Telephone: (800) 924-9897

This organization publishes a monthly newsletter as well as providing workshops and materials addressing vision needs in children and adults.

All About Vision Consumer Guide
Website: www.allaboutvision.com/

This website offers an extensive consumer guide on subjects relating to eye health, vision care, and learning disabilities.

American Occupational Therapy Association
4720 Montgomery Lane
P.O. Box 31220
Bethesda, MD 20824-1220
Telephone: (301) 652-2682
Website: www.aota.org/

This is the professional membership organization of occupational therapists. It provides public education and referrals for occupational therapy services.

Autism Independent UK
Website: www.autismuk.com/

This useful website offers many information resources for parents and professionals, including an extensive listing of links to worldwide websites relating to autism.

Autism Society of America
7910 Woodmont Avenue, Suite 300
Bethesda, MD 20814-3067
Telephone: (800) 328-8476
Website: www.autism-society.org/

This agency provides a range of information and referral services for children with autism.

CHADD National
8181 Professional Place, Suite 150
Landover, MD 20785
Telephone: (800) 233-4050
Website: www.chadd.org/

This organization sponsors support groups for parents of children with AD/HD, and provides continuing education programs for parents and professionals.

Children's Defense Fund
25 E. Street NW
Washington, DC 20001
Telephone: (202) 628-8787 or (800) 233-1200
Website: www.childrensdefense.org/

This agency provides information about legislation pertaining to child health, welfare, and education. It publishes a consumer guide describing parent rights under the Individuals with Disabilities Education Act.

Children's Vision Information Network
Website: www.childrensvision.com/

This is a useful website that offers excellent reviews of the relationship of vision to learning, including pages that discuss the effectiveness of vision therapy, and links to other related websites.

College of Optometrists in Vision Development

243 N. Lindbergh Boulevard, Suite 310
St. Louis, MO 63141
Telephone: (888) 268-3770
Website: www.covd.org/

This website offers extensive resource information for parents, teachers, and therapists, as well as a directory of qualified optometrists. It includes useful articles about the role of vision in autism, AD/HD, and learning disabilities.

Developmental Delay Resources

4401 East-West Highway, Suite 207
Bethesda, MD 20814
Telephone: (301) 652-2263 or (301) 652-9133
Website: www.devdelay.org/

This organization serves as a clearinghouse on alternative approaches to educational and medical treatment of children with special needs.

Educational Resources Information Center (ERIC) ERIC Clearinghouse on Disabilities and Gifted Education Council for Exceptional Children

1110 North Glebe Road, Suite 300
Arlington, VA 22201-5704
Telephone: (800) 328-0272 or Fax: (703) 264-9475
Website: http://ericec.org/

This is an association for parents and professionals with an interest in children with developmental differences. It provides literature reviews, referrals, and computer searches.

Future Horizons, Inc.

721 West Abram Street
Arlington, TX 76013
Telephone: (800) 489-0727
Website: www.futurehorizons-autism.com/

This organization offers extensive listings of publications and continuing education opportunities relating to autism. It also offers useful links to other autism-related websites.

Jessica Kingsley Publishers
116 Pentonville Road
London N1 9JB, UK
Telephone: (0)20 7833 2307
Website: www.jkp.com/

A publisher of accessible professional and academic books in the social and behavioral sciences, including a wide range of titles on developmental disabilities.

Learning Disabilities Association of America (LDA)
4156 Library Road
Pittsburgh, PA 15234-1349
Telephone: (412) 341-1515
Website: www.ldanatl.org/

This organization disseminates information, provides advocacy, and seeks to improve education opportunities for individuals with learning disabilities.

National Autistic Society
393 City Road
London EC1V 1NG, UK
Telephone: (0)20 7833 2299
Website: www.nas.org.uk/

This organization offers resources and services for children with autism and their families residing in the UK.

National Center for Learning Disabilities
381 Park Avenue South, Suite 1401
New York, NY 10016
Telephone: (212) 545-7510
Website: www.ncld.org/

This agency provides public awareness of learning disabilities by publishing a magazine for parents and professionals, and by providing computer-based information and referral services.

NetWellness Consumer Health Education
Website: www.netwellness.org/

This website partners with three leading universities to provide quality health care information on a variety of subjects, including vision and eye health care. It gives consumers the option of asking a personal question, which will be answered by an optometrist on faculty at one of the participating universities.

Optometric Extension Program
1921 E. Carnegie Avenue, Suite 3-L
Santa Ana, CA 92705-5510
Telephone: (949) 250-8070
Website: www.oep.org/

This website offers extensive articles and resources for parents and professionals, as well as an online store for books relating to vision and disabilities.

Optometrists Network
93 Bedford Street, Suite 5D
New York, NY 10014
Website: www.optometrists.org/

This website offers a directory of participating optometrists as well as useful articles for parents, therapists, and teachers. Links to other websites relating to learning disabilities and AD/HD are included. This site also contains some child-friendly pages that discuss vision difficulties and offers games and screening tests appropriate for older children, and a link to anecdotal reports from parents whose children have had success following vision therapy.

Publishers of tests for visual perception

Academic Therapy Publications
20 Commercial Boulevard
Novato, CA 94949-6191
Telephone: (800) 422-7249
Website: http://www.academictherapy.com/

American Guidance Services, Inc.
4201 Woodland Road
Circle Pines, MN 55014-1796
Telephone: (800) 328-2560
Website: www.agsnet.com/

Modern Curriculum Press
4350 Equity Drive
Columbus, OH 43216-2649
Telephone: (800) 321-3106
Website: www.plgcatalogue.pearson.com/

Pro-Ed, Inc.
8700 Shoal Creek Boulevard
Austin, TX 78757-6897
Telephone: (800) 897-3202
Website: www.proedinc.com/

Psychological Assessment Resources, Inc.
16204 N. Florida Avenue
Lutz, FL 33549
Telephone: (800) 331-8378 (USA)
Telephone: (813) 968-3003 ext. 361 (Canada)
Telephone: (0800) 092 3005 (UK)
Telephone: (1800) 101 607 (Australia)
Website: www.parinc.com/

Riverside Publishing
425 Spring Lake Drive
Itasca, IL 60143-2079
Telephone: (800) 323-9540
Website: www.riverpub.com/

Slosson Educational Publications, Inc.
P.O. Box 280
538 Buffalo Road
East Aurora, NY 14052-0280
Telephone: (888) 756-7766
Website: www.slosson.com/

Western Psychological Services
12031 Wilshire Boulevard
Los Angeles, CA 90025-1251
Telephone: (800) 648-8857 or (310) 478-2061
Website: www.wpspublish.com/

Suppliers of therapy and educational materials

Abilitations
3155 Northwoods Parkway
Norcross, GA 30071
Telephone: (800) 850-8602 or (770) 449-5700 (International)
Website: www.abilitations.com/

Childcraft Education Corporation
P.O. Box 3239
Lancaster, PA 17604
Telephone: (800) 631-5652
Website: www.childcrafteducation.com/

Flaghouse, Inc.
601 Flaghouse Drive
Hasbrouck Heights, NJ 07604-3116
Telephone: (800) 793-7900 or (201) 288-7600 (USA)
Telephone: (800) 265-6900 or (416) 495-8262 (Canada)
Website: www.flaghouse.com/

Funtastic Learning
206 Woodland Road
Hampton, NH 03842
Telephone: (800) 722-7375 or (603) 926-0071
Website: www.funtasticlearning.com/

OT Ideas, Inc.
124 Morris Turnpike
Randolph, NJ 07869
Telephone: (877) 768-4322 or (973) 895-3622
Website: www.otideas.com/

PDP Products
14524 61st Street Ct. N.
Stillwater, MN 55082
Telephone: (651) 439-8865
Website: www.pdppro.com/

Pocket Full of Therapy
P.O. Box 174
Morganville, NJ 07751
Telephone: (732) 441-0404
Website: www.pfot.com/

Primary Concepts
P.O. Box 10043
Berkeley, CA 94709
Telephone: (800) 660-8646
Website: www.primaryconcepts.com/

Southpaw Enterprises
P.O. Box 1047
Dayton, OH 45401
Telephone: (800) 228-1698 or (937) 252-7676 (International)
Website: www.southpawenterprises.com/

Therapro, Inc.
225 Arlington Street
Framingham, MA 01702-8723
Telephone: (800) 257-5376 or (508) 872-9494
Website: www.theraproducts.com/

Therapy Shoppe, Inc.
P.O. Box 8875
Grand Rapids, MI 49518
Telephone: (800) 261-5590 or (616) 696-7441
Website: www.therapyshoppe.com/

Toys to Grow On
2695 E. Dominguez St.
Carson, CA 90895
Telephone: (800) 987-4454
Website: www.toystogrowon.com/

EQUIPMENT FABRICATION

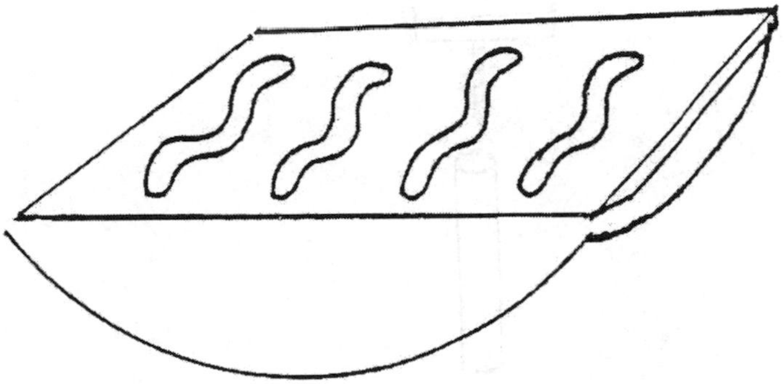

Figure A.1: Balance board

Balance board

Materials needed:

- 20" by 14" piece of plywood, $\frac{3}{4}$" thick
- Two 20" long by 3" maximum height curved pieces of plywood
- $1\frac{1}{2}$" wood nails
- Anti-slip bathtub treads (optional)

Assembly:

1. Sand edges of wood to prevent splinters.
2. Use nails to attach the wooden curves to the edges of the rectangle.
3. Apply treads to the top of the rectangle to prevent slipping (optional).

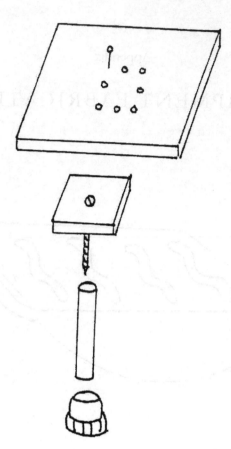

Figure A.2: Balance stool

One-legged balance stool

Materials needed:

- 8"square of plywood, $\frac{3}{4}$" thick
- 3" plywood square, $\frac{3}{4}$" thick
- Wooden dowel, 1" diameter by 8" long
- Eight 1" nails
- One $1\frac{1}{2}$" wood screw
- Rubber crutch tip (available at pharmacies or medical supply stores)

Assembly:

1. Sand edges of wood squares to prevent splinters.

2. Insert screw through 3" wood square into dowel.

3. Place large wood square over center of small square and secure using nails.

4. Place rubber crutch tip over bottom of dowel.

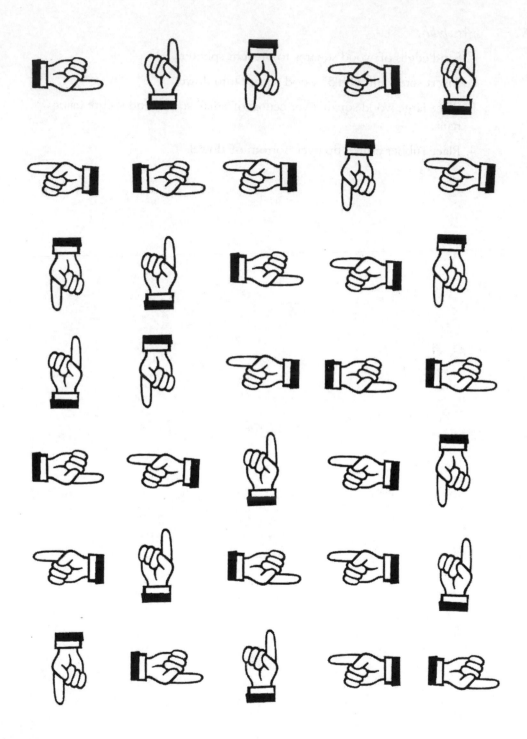

Figure A.3: Finger chart

Finger chart

Have the child stand on a balance beam or board and "read" the fingers as he or she follows each line of the chart from left to right. Older children can call out the direction of the fingers (left, right, up, down) while younger children can use their fingers to point in the same direction as the pictures.

GLOSSARY

Accommodation   The ability to change the shape of the lens by contracting the ciliary muscles so that the eye can change focus and see clearly from near and far.

Amblyopia   The loss of visual acuity due to disuse of the visual tract, as opposed to a refractive error or eye disease. Also known as *lazy eye*.

Anisometropia   A significant difference in refractive error between the two eyes.

Anophthalmia   A congenital malformation resulting in absence of the eyeball at birth.

Anterior chamber   The portion of the eye that is contained by the cornea in the front, and the iris in the back, containing the aqueous humor.

Aqueous humor   Clear fluid, mostly comprised of water, that fills the anterior and posterior chambers of the eye.

Astigmatism   A refractive error that is caused by an oval shape to the eyeball, which causes light rays entering the eye to focus at two different points. This causes blurring and distortion of vision at both near and far points.

Bilateral integration   The neurological process of organizing sensations from both sides of the body to allow coordinated movements between the two body sides.

Binocular vision   Ability of the two eyes to work together in order to simultaneously view the same object and create accurate depth perception. Also referred to as teaming.

Blindness   Legal blindness is defined as visual acuity of 20/200 or less in the better seeing eye using glasses, or a field of view that is narrower than 20°. Visual acuity of 20/70 or less in the better seeing eye using glasses is usually considered the criterion for eligibility to receive special education services in public schools.

Cataract   Opacity in the lens of the eye.

Choroid   Middle layer of the eye coverings (between the retina and the sclera) containing the blood vessels.

Ciliary body (muscle)   Circular muscle located behind the iris that is responsible for changing the shape of the lens.

Closure   See *visual closure*.

Conjunctiva   Mucous membrane covering the sclera and inner portions of the eyelids.

Conjunctivitis   Inflammation of the conjunctiva.

Convergence   The ability of the two eyes to come together to look at a near object. At its extreme, convergence is also known as crossed eyes.

Cornea   Clear, circular tissue that covers the anterior chamber of the eye, and is responsible for the refraction of light as it enters the eye.

Diopter   A unit of measure that indicates the strength of the refracting power of a lens.

Directionality   The ability to interpret directions such as right and left, up and down, in front and in back, etc.

Divergence	The ability of the eyes to move away from one another in order to focus on a distant object.
Emmetropia	Normal eyesight, with no refractive error.
Esophoria	A condition in which the eyes tend to turn inwards, but the person is able to control this tendency.
Esotropia	A form of strabismus in which the eyes tend to turn inwards and the person cannot control this tendency.
Eye hand coordination	The ability to use the eyes to monitor and guide the hand during motor activity.
Exophoria	A condition in which the eyes tend to turn outwards, but the person is able to control this tendency.
Exotropia	A form of strabismus in which the eyes tend to turn outwards and the person cannot control this tendency.
Farsightedness	See *hyperopia*.
Figure–ground discrimination	See *visual figure–ground discrimination*.
Form constancy	See *visual form constancy*.
Fovea	Central portion of the retina containing the cones, which allow fine vision of details and the recognition of color. The ability to use smooth, rapid eye movements allows a person to keep a visual target focused upon the fovea.
Fusion	The ability of the brain to coordinate images received by each of the eyes into a single image of the object.
Hemianopsia	Blindness in one-half of the visual field of one or both eyes, caused by damage to the optic nerve.

Hyperopia Farsightedness. The light rays entering the eyes focuses behind the retina, and the person must use muscular effort to accommodate in order to see clearly. The effort required is greatest when looking at very close objects. Blurred vision results when the person cannot accommodate sufficiently.

Hypertropia A form of strabismus in which the eyes tend to turn upwards and the person cannot control this tendency.

Iris The membrane located behind the cornea and in front of the lens, which creates the color of the eye.

Kinesthesia Knowledge of joint position and body movement in space, without the use of vision. For example, this would allow a person to be able to write their name in the air with eyes closed.

Laterality The ability to identify left and right on one's own body parts.

Lazy eye See *amblyopia*.

Lens A transparent and highly flexible structure located behind the iris and in front of the vitreous humor. It helps to bend light rays onto the retina.

Lenses Optical devices that are used to provide different visual experiences, such as helping the eyes to focus more clearly or relax focus.

Macula The central part of the retina dedicated to detail and color vision.

Myopia Nearsightedness. The light rays entering the eye are focused in front of the retina, resulting in blurred vision at a distance, but clear vision for close objects.

Near point of convergence	The point at which the eyes are in a position of maximum convergence, just before the person reports double vision. Normally, this should occur about two to four inches from the eyes.
Nearsightedness	See *myopia*.
Nystagmus	Involuntary, jerking movements of one or both eyes.
Occupational therapist	A licensed professional who is trained to evaluate the impact of disabilities on daily function, and to improve independence in daily occupational tasks through active involvement with purposeful activities. The role with children includes helping to evaluate and treat problems with visual perception, visual-motor integration, and fine motor control.
Ocular motility	See *ocular pursuits*.
Ocular pursuits	The ability to move the eyes to smoothly follow a moving target. Also referred to as visual pursuits, or visual tracking.
OD	Right eye (abbreviation for *oculus dexter*).
Ophthalmologist	A physician who specializes in the medical diagnosis and treatment of conditions of the eye, including surgery when indicated, and the prescription of glasses.
Optic chiasm	Location where some fibers from each optic nerve cross over to the opposite side of the brain. This allows each side of the brain to receive visual images from each eye.
Optic nerve	The nerve (Cranial nerve II) that carries neurological impulses from the eye to the brain.
Optometrist	A licensed clinician who specializes in evaluation and management of eye disorders, including the prescription of glasses.

Optometrist, developmental/ behavioral	An optometrist with advanced training who specializes in all aspects of a child's vision as related to the child's development and learning. In addition to prescribing glasses when indicated, this professional may also offer vision training to improve the child's functional use of vision.
OS	Left eye (abbreviation for *oculus sinister*).
OU	Both eyes (abbreviation for *oculus uterque*).
Photophobia	Excessive sensitivity to light.
Posterior chamber	The space located behind the iris and in front of the lens, that holds the aqueous humor.
Presbyopia	A refractive error caused by age-related decline in accommodative ability. People with this condition lose visual acuity at near point.
Proprioception	Body awareness that is obtained through various sensations coming from the joints, muscles, tactile receptors in the skin, and from gravity and motion.
Ptosis	Drooping of the eyelid.
Pupil	Opening in the central portion of the iris that allows light to travel to the back of the eye, visible as the dark circle in the center of the eyeball. The pupil opens wide in dark conditions, giving it a larger appearance, and narrows during conditions of bright light.
Pursuits	See *ocular pursuits*.
Refraction	The evaluation of visual acuity.
Retina	The most internal layer of the eye, that functions to organize incoming light signals, and changes these into electrical signals to be transmitted to the brain via the optic nerves.

Saccades   Eye movements used to shift rapidly from one target to another.

Sclera   A thick, protective covering of the eye that lies beneath the conjunctiva. This is recognized as the white part of the eye.

Sensory integration The neurological process of organizing sensory input in order to make an adaptive response for learning or behaving appropriately.

Stereopsis   Binocular visual perception of space, allowing perception of depth.

Strabismus   A condition in which the eyes are turned in some or all of the time. See also *esotropia*, *exotropia*, and *hypertropia*.

Suppression   A condition usually associated with strabismus and amblyopia in which the brain ignores the input from one eye.

Teaming   See *binocular vision*.

Vestibular   The sensory system, located within the inner ear, that provides information about gravity, body movement within space, and head position. This sense plays an important role in balance, posture, and coordinated movements of the eyes and body.

Vision therapy   Also referred to as orthoptics, vision training, or eye training. Vision therapy is undertaken by or under the guidance of an optometrist, and uses a wide variety of procedures to improve neuromuscular or neurophysiological vision dysfunction.

Visual acuity   Measurement of the clearness of vision, usually quantified as the smallest identifiable object visible at a distance of 20 feet. 20/20 is considered to be normal visual acuity.

Visual attention   A perceptual process involving alertness and readiness for learning through visual stimuli.

Visual closure	The ability to recognize forms or objects that are missing parts or are incompletely presented. Weakness in this perceptual skill often contributes to problems with spelling and reading comprehension.
Visual discrimination	A perceptual process involving the ability to recognize the basic features of visual stimuli, such as shape, size, orientation, or color.
Visual efficiency	The effectiveness of the visual system to see clearly and comfortably in order to achieve a quality of daily living. Component skills that are important in this process include accommodation, binocular vision, and ocular motility.
Visual figure–ground discrimination	Sometimes called figure–ground separation, this is the perceptual skill that allows the child to separate foreground from background visual stimuli in order to attend to the relevant details. Children with this problem may have difficulty attending when there are too many stimuli on a page, and may frequently lose their place. This is a common problem among children with AD/HD.
Visual form constancy	The perceptual ability to recognize that forms and objects remain the same even if they are seen in different environments or are slightly modified. It is this perceptual skill that enables the child to recognize the letter "A" whether it is in uppercase, lowercase, or cursive formation.
Visual memory	The ability to recall visually presented material. Immediate recall of information is sometimes referred to as working memory, while recall of the order of multiple stimuli is referred to as visual sequential memory.
Visual-motor integration	The ability to integrate visual information processing skills with motor movement, such as is needed to write or draw, catch a ball, or guide scissors to cut along a line. Also referred to as eye hand coordination.

Visual perception   Also referred to as visual analysis skills or visual cognitive skills. The ability to understand, interpret, and make use of visual information for cognitive problem solving. There are many different types of visual perception skills, including discrimination of shape, color, size; figure–ground separation; memory; closure; spatial awareness.

Visual sequential memory   See *visual memory*.

Visual-spatial perception   The perceptual ability to recognize the orientation and position of objects relative to one another and to oneself. This allows the child to recognize and develop the vocabulary for such concepts as left/right, up/down, in front/behind. Children who lack this perceptual skill frequently reverse letters, numbers and words far beyond the age where it is developmentally appropriate to do so.

Vitreous humor   Transparent gel, mostly composed of water, that fills the eyeball, holding the retina in place and providing support for the lens.

Working memory   See *visual memory*.

INDEX

Page numbers in *italic* refer to figures and tables.

accommodation 17–18, *18*, 30
AD/HD
  agencies and organizations 81–5
  and perceptual problems 48
  and vision disorders 12–13, 37–8
anatomy *see* visual system, anatomy
albinism 26
alignment, screening for 41
amblyopia 32
anopthalmia 26
astigmatism 29–30
attention deficit hyperactivity disorder *see* AD/HD
autism
  agencies and organizations 81–5
  and perceptual problems 48–9
  and vision disorders 12, 37

balance board, construction of *89*
balance stool, construction of *90*
Batshaw, M.L. *16*, *18*, *19*, *31*
Beery VMI *52*
Bender Visual-Motor Gestalt Test *52*
Benton Visual Retention Test *52*
binocular vision 17, 30–2
binocular vision disorders *see* strabismus; non-strabismic binocular vision disorders
Bouska, M.J. *43*

cataracts, congenital 26
Cohen, A. *43*
color blindness 26
compensation strategies for vision problems 76–8
Comprehensive Test of Visual Functioning *52*
cones *see* retina
convergence insufficiency
  description of 32
  screening for 41
cortical blindness 26
cover test for strabismus 42

cross-eyed *see* esotropia

developmental/behavioral optometrist
  directories and referral services 46–7
  role in assessment of visual perception problems *50*
  services provided 41–2
  specialized training for 41, 44
developmental pediatrician
  role in assessment of visual perception problems *50*
Developmental Test of Visual Perception *53*

Erhardt, R.P. *43*
Erhardt Developmental Vision Assessment *43*
esophoria 32
esotropia 31
exophoria 32
exotropia 31
extraocular muscles
  description of 17
  role in binocular vision 31–2

eye doctor
    choosing a specialist 42,
        44–7
    directories and referral
        programs 46–7
    see also developmental/
        behavioral
        optometrist;
        ophthalmologist;
        optometrist
eye hand coordination see
    visual-motor integration

farsightedness see hyperopia
figure–ground
    discrimination see visual
        figure–ground
        discrimination
form constancy see visual
    form constancy
form perception see visual
    discrimination
fovea see retina
functional vision
    impairments
    categories of 28
    clinical screening for 41–2
    screening tests 43
    suggested activities 62–70

glaucoma, congenital 26

hemianopsia 26–7
hyperopia 28–9
hyperphoria 32
hypertropia 31

intervention for visual
    problems
    activities to improve
        functional vision
        62–70
    activities to improve
        visual perception
        70–4
    desirable qualities of an
        intervention program
        58
    general guidelines 61–2
    role of parents 57
    suppliers of therapy and
        educational material
        86–8

Jordan Left/Right Reversal
    Test 53

Kaufman, N. 43
Kaufman Assessment
    Battery for Children 53
Kent Visual Perceptual Test
    53

lazy eye see amblyopia
learning disabilities
    agencies and
        organizations 81–5
    and perceptual problems
        48
    and vision disorders
        12–13, 37
Leber's amaurosis 27
Lieberman, S. 43

macula see retina
macular degeneration 27
Marcus, S.E. 43
McDowell, P.M. 43
McDowell, R.L. 43
McDowell Vision Screening
    Kit 43
memory see visual memory
Motor-Free Visual
    Perception Test 53
myopia 28

nearsightedness see myopia
Neitz Test of Color Vision
    53
NEPSY®: A Developmental
    Neuropsychological
    Assessment 53
neurologist
    role in assessment of
        visual perception
        problems 50
neuropsychologist
    role in assessment of
        visual perception
        problems 50
non-strabismic binocular
    vision disorders 32
nurse
    role in vision screening 41
NYSOA Vision Battery 43

occupational therapist
    description of 49, 52
    role in assessment of
        visual perception
        problems 50–1
    role in vision screening 41

ocular motility disorders 32–3

ocular tracking
screening for 41
see also ocular motility disorders

ophthalmologist
description of 42

optic nerve
atrophy 27
hypoplasia 27

optic pathways see visual system, anatomy

optometrist
description of 42, 44
directories and referral programs 46–7
see also developmental/ behavioral optometrist

Pediatric Clinical Vision Screening for Occupational Therapists 43

phoria 32

presbyopia 30

Preschool Visual Motor Integration Assessment 53

proprioceptive system 63–4

psychologist
role in assessment of visual perceptual problems 51

reading specialist
role in assessment of visual perceptual problems 51

refractive errors of vision see astigmatism; hyperopia; myopia

retina 17

retinitis pigmentosa 27

retinopathy of prematurity 27

Richards, R.G. 43

Ritty, M. 43

rods see retina

saccades
description of 32
screening for 41

Scheiman, M. 43

school psychologist see psychologist

sensory integration therapy 49

Sensory Integration and Praxis Tests (SIPT) 54

spatial perception see visual-spatial perception

special educator
role in assessment of visual perceptual problems 51

standardized tests of visual perception see tests

Stanford-Binet Intelligence Scales 54

Stolzber, M. 43

strabismus
cover test 42
description of 31–2
see also hyperopia; esotropia; exotropia

suppression 32

Test of Visual-Perceptual Skills (non-motor) 54

tests of visual perception
American laws governing testing in schools 55–7
choosing appropriate tests 52–5
publishers of 85–6
understanding test scores 56

vestibular sense 63

vision
development in infants 21–3
development in toddlers and preschoolers 23–4
relationship to developing motor control 62–4
relationship to learning 11, 21
relationship to social skills 24

vision disorders
and AD/HD 12–13, 37–8
and autism 12, 37
and eligibility for special education 55–7
and learning disabilities 12–13, 37
compensatory strategies 76–8
functional vision disorders 28–33
incidence of 12, 37
structural vision disorders 25–7
symptoms of 13, 38–40
visual efficiency disorders 30–3
see also visual perception

vision problem *see* vision
 disorder
vision therapy
 effectiveness of 45
 services provided 44–5
visual acuity
 description of 28
 screening for 41
visual attention 33
visual closure 33
visual cognition *see* visual
 perception
visual discrimination
 activities to improve 71
 description of 34
visual figure–ground
 discrimination
 activities to improve 71–2
 description of 34
visual form constancy 34
visual hygiene
 activities to improve 75–6
 relationship to daily living
 skills 75
visual information
 processing *see* visual
 perception
visual memory
 activities to improve 73
 description of 34
visual-motor integration
 34–5
visual perception
 activities to improve 70–4
 assessment of 48–56
 description of 33, 48
 problems with 33–5
 tests 52–4
Visual Skills Appraisal *43*

visual-spatial perception
 activities to improve 72–4
 description of 35
visual system, anatomy
 extraocular muscles 17, 31
 eye 15–18
 general structure 15, *16*
 optic pathways 18–19
 retina 17
visual tracking *see* ocular
 tracking

wall-eyed *see* exotropia
Wechsler Intelligence Scale
 for Children *54*
Wide Range Assessment of
 Memory and Learning
 54